P9-EJU-083

# DROPPING ACID

# DROPPING ACID
## THE REFLUX DIET
### COOKBOOK & CURE

Dropping Acid: The Reflux Diet Cookbook & Cure

Copyright © 2010 The Reflux Cookbooks, LLC, a division of Katalitix Media
ISBN: 978-0-9827083-1-6
Printed in the United States of America by G & H Soho, Inc. (Elmwood Park, NJ)

7th Printing, November 2016

All rights reserved. No part of this publication may be reproduced or transmitted in any form or by any means, electronic or mechanical, including photocopying, recording, or any other storage and retrieval system, without the express written permission of Dr. Jamie Koufman (www.KoufmanReflux.com).

**Notice and Disclaimer**

This book is intended as a reference volume only, not as a medical manual. The information given here is designed to help you make informed decisions about your health. It is not intended as a substitute for any treatment that might have been prescribed by your doctor. If you suspect that you have a medical problem, we urge you to seek medical help. Any use of this book is at the reader's discretion, as the advice and strategies contained within may not be suitable for every individual.

Mention of specific companies, organizations, or authorities in this book does not imply endorsement by the authors or the publisher, nor does mention of specific companies, organizations, or authorities imply that they endorse this book.

Measurements of acidity (pH) of the foods and beverages listed in this book were done by the authors using a Minilab ISFET pH meter (Model IQ128 pH meter with Silicon Chip Sensor, Pulse Instruments, Carlsbad, CA). The pH meter was calibrated before each use and cleaned between measurements, and it was noted that the device returned to neutral pH before taking the next measurement. Nevertheless, we recognize that sampling error can occur, and that any particular measurement might show significant variance. In addition, a particular food item can vary significantly in pH from day to day and from batch to batch, and depending on ripeness, growing conditions, handling, and processing.

*Designed by:* Rogers Seidman Design
*All photographs in this book were taken by Jamie Koufman and Jordan Stern.*

***Cover:*** Crunchy Cucumber and Fennel Salad (page 90); photo by Jordan Stern.
*Note:* The green sliced vegetables in the dish are sliced green beans, not jalapeño peppers. There are no jalapeños in **The Reflux Diet.**

*Dedicated to our patients*
*who asked for this book*

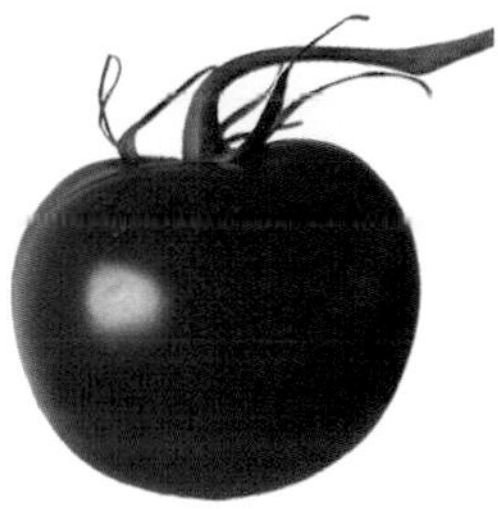

“I have never developed indigestion from eating my words.”
Winston Churchill

“I saw few die of hunger; of eating, a hundred thousand.”
Benjamin Franklin

“It’s difficult to think anything but pleasant thoughts
while eating a homegrown tomato.”
Lewis Grizzard

# Contents

11 | Preface
15 | The Accidental Chefs

THE CURE

21 | What You Eat Could Be Eating You
31 | How Do I Know If I Have Reflux?
37 | Maintaining Health: The Reflux Cure

THE DIET

45 | Getting Started on the Reflux Diet
49 | Best Foods for a Refluxer
55 | Notoriously Bad Reflux Foods
61 | Avoiding Acidic Foods and Beverages
65 | Delicious Low-Fat Cooking

THE COOKBOOK

70 | Breakfast
87 | Salads
100 | Soups
109 | Entrées (Lunch & Dinner)
131 | Hors d'Oeuvres & Snacks
140 | Desserts

THE SCIENCE

159 | Reflux Science You Can Digest by Jamie A. Koufman, M.D.
177 | References
187 | Acidity (pH) of Common Foods and Beverages

192 | About the Authors
195 | Acknowledgments
196 | Index

# Preface

Acid reflux is epidemic, and you probably don't even know you have it.

Do you cough or clear your throat a lot after eating a meal? Wake up in the middle of the night coughing or short of breath? Is your throat hoarse or sore in the morning? Do you have the sensation of a lump in your throat, or difficulty swallowing? Are you plagued by postnasal drip?

*Reflux is not just indigestion and heartburn.* We now know about "silent reflux"—a term coined by Dr. Jamie Koufman—in which you may experience many of the above symptoms *without* indigestion.

**Dropping Acid: The Reflux Diet Cookbook & Cure** is the first book to acknowledge that reflux comes in many colors—a concept that is just now coming to the public's attention. If you are over forty, there's a 50/50 chance you already have it. Reflux is one of the most important, misunderstood, and preventable diseases of Western civilization. **We estimate that 100 million Americans have reflux, many of them unaware of it, and many of them incorrectly diagnosed.**

Not only is reflux amazingly widespread, its incidence is on the rise. Why? *We believe it has largely to do with excessive acid in our diets.*

You see, it's not just about obesity and overeating, as many people think. Reflux increasingly strikes the thin, the athletic . . . *and the young.* A generation ago, almost all the reflux patients we saw were in their 40s and 50s; today, they're as likely to be in their 20s and 30s. Dr. Jamie Koufman remembers a patient who had just graduated from NYU with her heart set on becoming a Broadway star, but whose perpetual hoarseness was interfering with her singing. She was only 21, but it was already so far gone that she needed surgery. Perhaps more disturbing was that all her friends were experiencing the same symptoms! They're not the first generation of college grads to go out for a beer on a Saturday night, but they're the first generation to pay for it so dearly.

Not only are we seeing reflux in a younger population, we're seeing less of the classic symptom of heartburn and more of the symptoms listed at the start of this chapter. Reflux is changing and adapting with the times, and so must we.

**Reflux is complicated.** It makes certain foods your enemy. The symptoms that are stirred up by late-night eating can affect your sleep, and poor sleep eats away at quality of life and other aspects of your health.

**Reflux is pernicious.** We believe it is a major cause of cancer of the esophagus and throat, and possibly other cancers as well.

Fortunately, for many people there is a cure. It is right here in this cookbook, where two doctors take everything they know about reflux and join forces with a creative chef.

*But this is not just a cookbook.* We certainly hope you will prepare and enjoy the delicious, healthful dishes French Master Chef Marc Bauer developed for this book using cutting-edge medical research on foods that are "safe," but we also encourage you to read the chapters on the science behind reflux, where we explain what causes reflux and its symptoms, and why this poses such a serious health risk for you.

In part, we present and explain the science because we realize how controversial reflux has become, with many points of view on it tied to many different and segmented medical specialties. As experts in the field for a long time, we have worked conscientiously to provide a fair and accurate overview of a most misunderstood condition. In the chapter "What You Eat Could Be Eating You" (page 21), we explain reflux in terms anyone can understand. If you're of a more scientific bent, the chapter "Reflux Science You Can Digest" (page 159) presents a more comprehensive and documented account of the medical research—much of it done by Dr. Jamie Koufman—that helps fill the gap between reflux as it may be understood by your local doctor and reflux as it affects your everyday life.

The research in this book lends scientific validity and authority to the sensible health concerns of those consumers, organizations, and political leaders who are interested in monitoring the quality and safety of our food. By reading one or both of the science chapters, you will better understand why and how the recipes in **Dropping Acid: The Reflux Diet Cookbook & Cure** can help you feel well and get healthier . . . not just when you're in need of a quick fix, but for good.

re·flux *n* [ L *re-* back + *fluxus* flow ]
1: a flowing back 2: a process of refluxing

## COMMON TERMS FOR REFLUX

### General Terms

Acid reflux

Gastric reflux

Indigestion

Heartburn

### Terms for Esophageal Reflux

Gastroesophageal reflux disease (GERD)

Gastro-oesophageal reflux disease (GORD) [U.K.]

Peptic esophagitis / Esophageal erosions

### Terms for Throat Reflux

Laryngopharyngeal reflux (LPR)

Extraesophageal reflux disease

Supraesophageal reflux disease

Atypical reflux disease

Reflux laryngitis

SIlent reflux

Airway reflux

# The Accidental Chefs

This book came about through a combination of friendship and common purpose. Two of the authors are medical doctors (trained as ear, nose, and throat specialists), and the third is a master chef. Drs. Jamie Koufman and Jordan Stern were urged to write this book by their reflux patients, for whom the standard two-page brochure wasn't enough to help them figure out what to eat on a daily basis. French Master Chef Mark Bauer was interested in making his delicious cuisine accessible to patrons with reflux.

When we set out to write this book, we already had experience treating thousands of patients with reflux. We knew all about the notorious bad-for-reflux foods. We knew that some foods cause reflux by disabling esophageal defenses, the equivalent of springing open a trap door.

We also knew that *acidic foods cause reflux symptoms.* This last point is a recent discovery, and the key to **The Reflux Diet.**

Reflux management has traditionally been about minimizing the impact of acid from the stomach below, but our research and clinical experience taught us

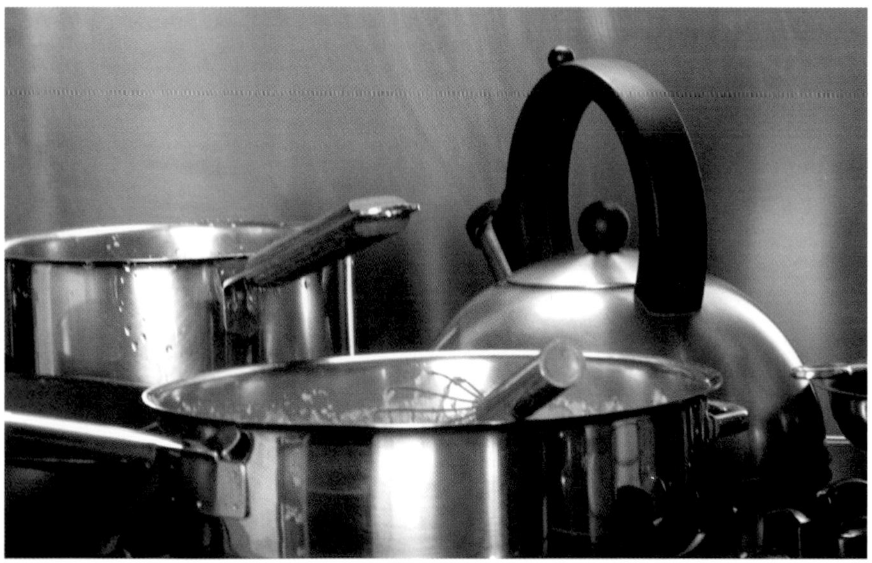

to be just as concerned with acid "from above." We found that for many reflux patients, a diet that was too acidic was just as bad as having continual gastric reflux, i.e., acid coming up from the stomach.

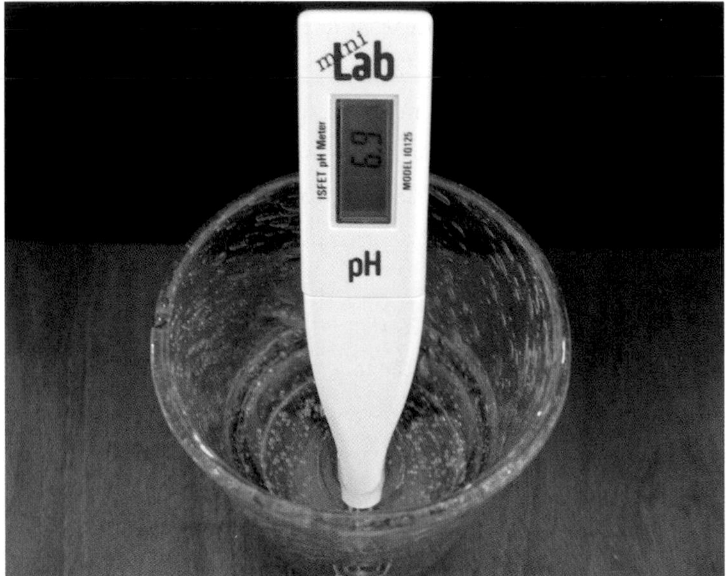


We tested the acidity of many foods and beverages using an ISFET pH Meter.

As a result, **The Reflux Diet Cookbook & Cure** offers new ideas about healthful eating and cooking. *This is the first diet cookbook to systematically address the problem of dietary acid.*

The authors talked, cooked, and ate their way through every recipe in this book, and we believe that our collaboration honestly reflects the state of the medical art and our combined years of experience.

Be prepared to consider some new ideas. Whole-grain breads, for example, are very good for avoiding reflux, and a slice or two makes a great snack. *Just remember that almost everything we recommend is going to be bad for someone, somewhere.* That's the way it is in the world of reflux. Oatmeal and bananas are great items for most refluxers, but not all. We welcome questions, suggestions, and recipes; you can add your comments, etc., to our blog at www.refluxcookbookblog.com.

**Dropping Acid: The Reflux Diet Cookbook & Cure** has been a work in progress for 25 years. That's because the principles and recommendations here have evolved as a direct result of clinical and basic medical science research. Until recently, no one understood enough about how reflux causes symptoms and diseases to counsel patients on exactly what to eat and what not to eat.

Naturally, there are foods you will have to learn to avoid. Barbecued ribs, French fries, and chocolate cake will never make a good meal for a refluxer. Still, we felt that the conventional antireflux diet was overly restrictive and focused only on what you *couldn't* eat—no fried food, no chocolate, no soda—so we came up with recipes that expanded on what you *could* eat. Wait till you try our oatmeal-crusted salmon!

**The Reflux Diet Cookbook & Cure** integrates science, medicine, and culinary art in a bold way. And while the focus of the book is self-directed reflux management, the basic principles are more broadly beneficial. When you maintain this way of eating, you also lose weight and become leaner and fitter—because these dishes are low in fat. In the past, "low fat" meant "no fat," leading to food with no taste. *Chef Bauer's idea to use tasty fats as flavorings, not as main ingredients, represents a paradigm shift in reflux cooking.*

**The Reflux Diet Cookbook & Cure** offers a healthy dietary foundation on which you can build. Our recipes are original, healthful, and delicious. They make good sense. And given that reflux-related esophageal cancer is currently one of the fastest-growing cancers in the U.S., this diet just might save your life.

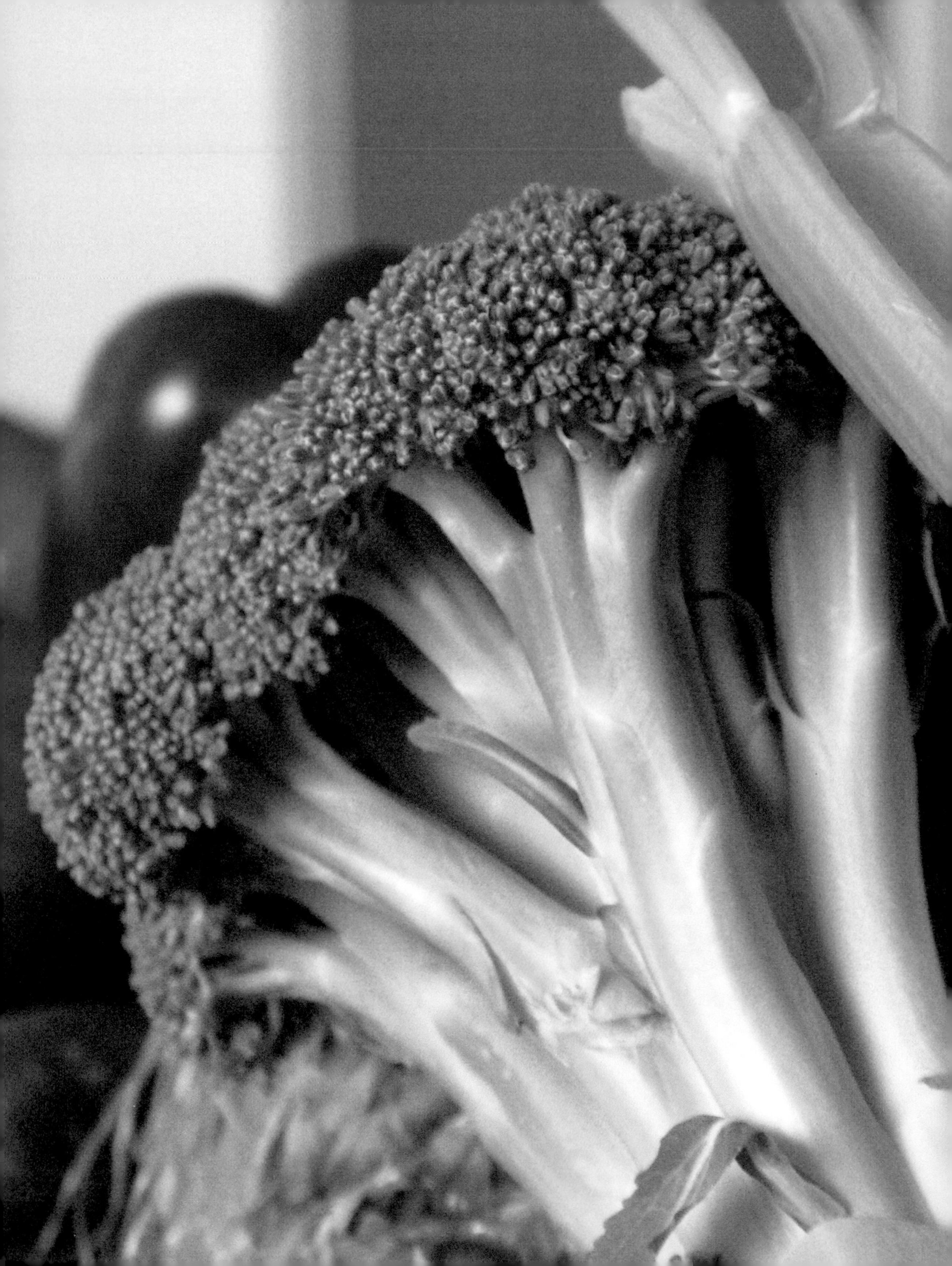

# *the* cure

# What You Eat Could Be Eating You

**Almost everyone has some reflux,** the upward backflow of the stomach's contents. Managing it will always require thought, creativity, and attention to what you eat and when. There's no one-size-fits-all strategy for beating it.

This chapter describes the science behind reflux in a way that will help you understand how and why **The Reflux Diet** works. To understand it further, the chapter "Reflux Science You Can Digest" later in this book (page 159) contains a more in-depth look at the scientific state of the art and research in this field, including many of the relevant references from the medical literature.

## Things Are Not What They Seem

Acid reflux has been poorly understood until recently, even by doctors in closely related fields. For example, your family doctor or even a specialist might have told you that it's asthma, sinusitis, or an allergy, when in fact you had reflux. Or perhaps your doctor prescribed an over-the-counter antacid. The real villain, however, is the digestive enzyme *pepsin,* not acid, so an antacid therefore won't do a thing for many reflux symptoms. At present, there is no "antipepsin" medication, so the disease that is literally eating away at you keeps on going.

Why should you care? *Because reflux is not only uncomfortable and inconvenient, it's dangerous.* If left untreated, reflux can wreak havoc on your throat, airways, lungs, and digestive system. It can even cause cancer.

The American diet has changed dramatically since WWII, but there has been no captain steering the ship—no overarching body to monitor all aspects of the safety of the food supply. This may explain why reflux and many reflux-related diseases are increasing in America.

Here's what happened. In the 1960s and 1970s, fast food and prepackaged food became popular, and many people stopped eating home-cooked meals.

In general, the obesity epidemic has paralleled the increase in the saturated fat content of our diets, but there has been a second, more insidious trend: *Prepared foods have been increasingly acidified* to prevent bacterial growth and add shelf life. Today, many prepared foods and beverages are just as acidic as stomach acid itself.

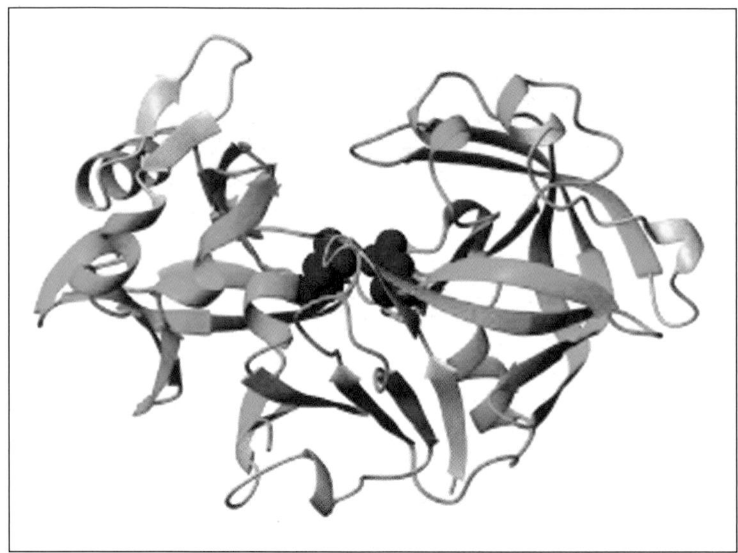

Computer-generated image of the human pepsin molecule. Pepsin is the principal digestive enzyme of the stomach, and it (not acid) is responsible for the tissue damage caused by reflux. Peptides were used to make antibodies for pepsin assays, which form the basis for new, noninvasive tests for reflux; see www.VoiceInstituteofNewYork.com. Dr. Jamie Koufman is the inventor of these diagnostic methods (US Patent No. 5,879,897).

*Until this book, no one has investigated the adverse effects of too much acid in the foods and beverages we consume.* Everyone worries about equalizing the stomach's natural acid, yet we continue to pour ever more acidified foods and drinks into it. Again, it's not stomach acid that's the main problem. The term "acid reflux" is misleading, since it is the digestive enzyme *pepsin,* not acid, that causes most of the trouble. The confusion is because pepsin can only do its job when acid is around to activate it. Then it gets busy breaking down proteins into smaller, more easily digestible particles. Without acid to supercharge it, pepsin can't do its thing.

Here's the catch: At a certain point, pepsin doesn't go away meekly after digesting your meal. It's still hanging around like the bully at a playground. All it needs is some acid to wake it up again. Your stomach produces acid when you eat a meal, but pepsin doesn't care *where* the acid comes from; any acid will do. Any foods you eat that are high in acid are perfectly sufficient for activating pepsin, and if there's no protein around that needs digesting, the pepsin will gnaw on whatever is handy—such as the linings of your throat and esophagus. The old adage "You are what you eat" might in this case be rephrased: "Be careful what you eat, because what you eat could be eating you."

Imagine that your stomach is full of seawater and lobsters. The seawater is acid, and the lobsters (big, aggressive ones with mighty claws) are the pepsin molecules. When you reflux, the seawater splashes around. Some of it splashes upward into your throat. The lobsters ride this wave of seawater and attach themselves to the shore wherever they land—the shore being the delicate tissue and membranes lining your throat, larynx (voice box), esophagus, and lungs.

The lobsters are hanging on by their claws. It doesn't really matter now whether the seawater they need for survival splashes up from below or pours down from above. To these lobsters, it's all just a delicious, rejuvenating splash. Once a pepsin molecule is bound to, say, your throat, *any* dietary source of acid can reactivate it: Soda pop. Salsa. Strawberries.

The pH scale, used to measure acidity, is somewhat counterintuitive. pH 7 is neutral; pH 1 is very acidic, and caustics like bleach have values from pH 8-14. For example, distilled water and most tap water is pH 7 (neutral), but vinegar at pH 2.9 and lemon juice at pH 2.7 are acidic. The normal range of stomach acid is pH 1-4. Also note that the pH scale is a logarithmic scale, so pH 4 is ten times more acidic than pH 5, and pH 4.8 is twice as acidic as 5.0. That's why simply diluting acidic beverages doesn't make them nonacidic.

We suspect that **Dropping Acid: The Reflux Diet Cookbook & Cure** will not be popular with federal regulatory agencies or the Congress that funds them. Or with some of the companies that produce commercial foods and beverages, because **many common products are as acidic as stomach acid and just as potentially harmful.** The acidification of prepackaged foods and beverages extends their shelf life and discourages bacterial growth, which is good. But it is also likely that this acidification of our food is one of the reasons reflux is approaching epidemic levels.

This book might also irritate certain members of the medical community. After all, different medical specialties have different perspectives. However, the prevailing clinical model of reflux disease is about as wrong as the ancient belief that the world is flat.

For one thing, there is a huge misconception about how pepsin works. Many doctors mistakenly believe that pepsin is only active below pH 4. Nothing could be further from the truth. Pepsin, that lobster, can continue to be somewhat active up to pH 6.

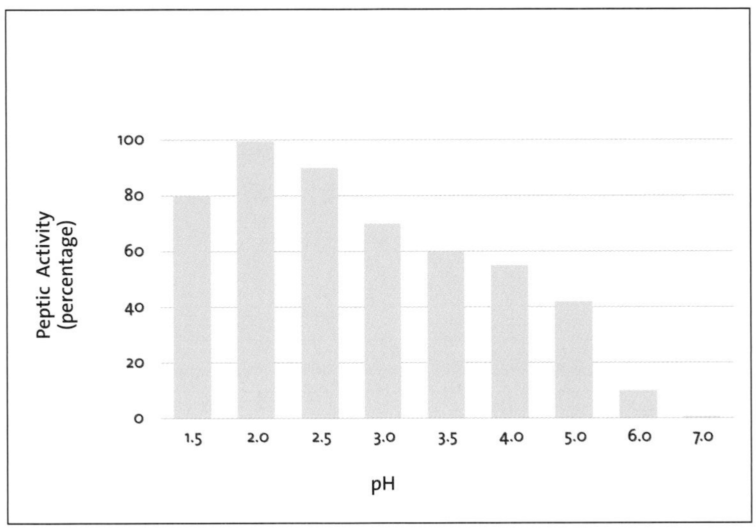


The old thinking was that pepsin wasn't active above pH 4, but this chart shows just how wrong that is. *(Reference: Johnston N, et al. Activity/stability of human pepsin: Implications for reflux-attributed laryngeal disease. Laryngoscope 117:1036-9, 2007.)*

Pepsin does maximum damage at pH 2 (100 percent activity), but it can still do some damage up to pH 6 (10 percent activity). This pepsin activation curve has important implications for reflux, because protein can be digested—and tissue damaged—to some degree *whenever any acid is present.* (In case you were wondering, Coca-Cola is pH 2.8.)

When pepsin binds to tissue, it remains stable for a long time. The question is not whether it is active, but *how* active. All those popular and expensive antireflux medicines don't actually *turn off* the acid; they just *turn it down,* reduce it somewhat. On television ads, you'll see those little acid pumps in the stomach give up at the sight of a powerful purple pill, but that's not what really happens. Even after taking the strongest antireflux medications, the *proton pump inhibitors* (e.g., Prilosec, Protonix, Nexium), everyone's stomach still churns out significant amounts of acid. About 10 percent of people who try proton pump inhibitors do not respond to them, and another 15–20 percent get side effects such as nausea, gas, bloating, diarrhea, and abdominal pain. Long-term use of PPIs (over years) appears to increase one's risk of developing esophageal cancer.

We still don't have a universally effective antireflux medication. The best medications we have are only pretty good, and they're only pretty good for about two-thirds of the people who need them.

By now you're probably wondering: "Why not forget the acid and just treat the pepsin?"

There is not yet an effective antipepsin medication. **However, what has been missing from the treatment equation until now is an understanding of the profound impact of dietary acid.** To correct this misunderstanding, here is a summary of exactly how reflux causes problems for you, the sufferer:

- Acid and pepsin work together to cause reflux-related symptoms and diseases.
- None of the available antireflux medications turn acid off completely.
- When pepsin attaches to human tissue, disease may result.
- Dietary acid can activate pepsin already in or on tissue.
- Tissue that is sick from reflux needs a period of recovery.

## Why Doesn't My Doctor Know About This?

Patients frequently ask us, "Why doesn't my doctor know about this?" Part of the answer is that specialists are too specialized. Many reflux symptoms (hoarseness, the sensation of a lump in the throat, postnasal drip, chronic throat clearing, cough, chest pain) cross medical specialty lines and are nonspecific. The correct diagnosis is often confused with other diagnoses, including upper respiratory infections, allergies, and sinusitis.

Patients with reflux-related chronic cough, for example, often see a number of physicians without receiving proper diagnosis and treatment; see chronic-

### From the Case Files of Dr. Koufman

*A respiratory therapist I treated in North Carolina was a big man: six foot four, 280 pounds. Even his voice was big, but it was always hoarse in the morning. At 38, he was keeping that weight up by chowing down on his favorites—grits and a half-pound of bacon for breakfast, fried chicken almost daily. In fact, he divided his patronage equally among the four big chicken chains: K&W Cafeteria, KFC, Church's, and Popeye's. You don't get to be 280 pounds for nothing.*

*I helped him, but this was a very sad case because he had left California to become a respiratory therapist only after his promising career as an opera singer fizzled. That career, it turned out, had been destroyed by something as simple (and as complicated, too) as reflux. He never knew what the problem was with his hoarse voice and was never properly diagnosed, so he abandoned a career he loved.*

*I stopped his late-night food binges and all-fried diet, and I sent him to a gym. The morning hoarseness cleared up, and he got his weight down to 215 pounds. He actually went back to singing, but it was too late for a professional career in opera.*

*By the way, you should not be waking up hoarse. It's not natural! In general, voice problems get worse as the day goes on, so if you're starting the morning with hoarseness or a sore throat, it probably means you're a nighttime refluxer.*

cough.net. They might find a knowledgeable specialist only after browsing the Internet and stumbling across information about "silent reflux," also known as *laryngopharyngeal reflux* (LPR). These frustrated patients may find relief only after being disappointed by visits to doctors in otolaryngology, allergy, immunology, gastroenterology, and pulmonary and internal medicine.

**Remember, what makes silent reflux insidious and difficult to diagnose is that people who have it DO NOT have heartburn and indigestion.** To most people (and their doctors), reflux and heartburn are synonymous, so they miss the big picture.

Silent reflux has much in common with other relatively recent medical discoveries that were at first misunderstood, but it is time to give silent reflux its due. It is the most important disease of the breathing passages, and it contributes to the development of many diseases of the ear, nose, throat, lungs, and esophagus—including the development of cancer. **At present, reflux-related esophageal cancer (most common in white males) is the fastest-growing cancer in the United States.** In addition, research on the cell biology of LPR has shown that laryngeal cancer and reflux exhibit similar cell damage profiles.

*We, the authors, believe that reflux may be one of the most important risk factors for the development of both esophageal and laryngeal cancers.*

**ELEMENTS OF THE REFLUX DIET**

1. Begin with two weeks on a very strict, acid-free diet (The Induction Reflux Diet). (See "Getting Started on the Reflux Diet," page 45.)
2. In the third week, go to the "maintenance" phase of the diet by choosing your foods and beverages from the "good" and "bad" food lists on pages 62–64.
3. Eat smaller meals more frequently, instead of large meals.
4. Do not eat anything three hours before bedtime.

## Principles of The Reflux Diet

As it turns out, the story of acid and pepsin (the main digestive enzyme of the stomach) makes a compelling case for a new approach to reflux management.

First, as you might have guessed, we recommend that you limit your intake of acidic foods and beverages, which we will describe and list later in this book.

Second, there are foods that cause reflux in an entirely different way from the lobsters-in-seawater analogy. These foods relax the stomach valve that normally keeps things down there from backflowing (refluxing) upward. That valve is called the *lower esophageal sphincter* (LES), and it can temporarily relax, or loosen, in the presence of the chemical composition of such foods as chocolate, caffeine, alcohol, and many high-fat delicacies, from fried foods to fatty meats.

Third, there are foods that increase pressure inside the stomach, resulting in a backflow that overcomes the LES valve. This group of foods and beverages includes anything that expands in the stomach, such as carbonated beverages (beer and soda).

By design, **The Reflux Diet** has two levels: (1) *induction (start-up)* and (2) *maintenance.* For the first two weeks, we recommend a very strict diet. We call this start-up period the *induction reflux diet* or *"pepsin washout" phase.* The idea is to give the membranes lining your throat, esophagus, etc., a chance to heal.

Next is the *maintenance diet,* which is less strict and can be sustained for a lifetime.

One final observation for newly diagnosed refluxers: It may take a year or more for you to acquire an understanding of all the variables that make your reflux better or worse. Try to be patient with the process. Reflux is generally intermittent anyway, so you'll have plenty of time to experiment. You will, however, have to change the way you think. From now on, you will always need to focus on what you eat and when. No more snacks on autopilot!

**The Reflux Diet Cookbook & Cure** is intended to help people with reflux, not to be a substitute for medical treatment. That said, there is no question that for many people with reflux, diet and lifestyle change is the key to successful treatment. Here are a few other steps you can take to reduce reflux and bring some relief:

- If you use tobacco, quit. *Smoking causes reflux.*
- Don't wear clothing that is too tight, especially trousers, corsets, bras, and belts.
- Avoid exercising right after eating (especially weightlifting, jogging, and yoga).
- Do not lie down right after eating, and do not eat within three to four hours of bedtime. Late-night eating is the number-one lifestyle risk factor for reflux.
- Elevate the head of your bed if you're a nighttime refluxer—that is, if you have symptoms of hoarseness, sore throat, or coughing in the morning.

The recipes in this book have been created as a welcome change from the tasteless reflux foods of the past and as the cornerstone of a healthy, sustainable diet. The nutritional profile of **The Reflux Diet** is an extension of the "healthy heart" diet, so we have no trouble recommending this diet to everyone. If, for example, you share your life with someone who has reflux, you could do worse than to cook and eat together according to **The Reflux Diet Cookbook & Cure.**

## From the Case Files of Dr. Koufman

*One patient flew in from Japan to see me. At 60, his singing career had been up and down over the years because of chronic cough. When I first looked at his larynx, I saw that, in addition to reflux, he had candida laryngitis—a furry fungus coating his esophagus and larynx.*

*He was not doing well. He couldn't perform. I treated the fungus and the reflux, but when I found out this man seemed to eat almost nothing but cherries, I also put him on* ***The Reflux Diet.*** *Today, he is again giving master classes in singing and has stopped coughing entirely for the first time in 35 years.*

# How Do I Know If I Have Reflux?

People with typical gastroesophageal reflux disease (GERD) have heartburn—chest pain after eating, particularly after eating fried or greasy foods. Most of the time, a doctor makes the diagnosis of GERD. The more difficult question is how to know if you have "atypical" or "silent" reflux, also called *laryngopharyngeal reflux* (LPR).

**COMMON SYMPTOMS OF REFLUX**

Hoarseness
Chronic cough
Choking episodes
Trouble swallowing
A lump in the throat
Chronic throat clearing
Postnasal drip
Heartburn
Asthma

LPR can occur during the day or night, but most people with LPR do not have heartburn. (Hence, "silent reflux.") The explanation for this is that refluxed material does not stay in the esophagus long enough to irritate that organ; however, if even a little of those stomach juices come up into the throat, symptoms can occur. Compared to the esophagus, the throat and voice box are a hundred times more sensitive to irritation and damage from reflux.

The symptoms of LPR are hoarseness, too much throat mucus, throat clearing, postnasal drip, chronic cough, a sensation of a lump in the throat, sore throat, choking episodes, shortness of breath, asthma, sinus problems, difficulty swallowing, dental disease, and even halitosis. Some people have intermittent or chronic hoarseness, while others have problems with too much nose and throat

## THE REFLUX SYMPTOM INDEX (RSI)

### Circle 0–5 in each of the 9 rows and add up the numbers to get your RSI

| How do the following affect you? | 0 = No Problem | | | 5 = Severe Problem | | |
|---|---|---|---|---|---|---|
| Hoarseness or a problem with your voice | 0 | 1 | 2 | 3 | 4 | 5 |
| Clearing your throat | 0 | 1 | 2 | 3 | 4 | 5 |
| Excess throat mucus or postnasal drip | 0 | 1 | 2 | 3 | 4 | 5 |
| Difficulty swallowing food, liquids, or pills | 0 | 1 | 2 | 3 | 4 | 5 |
| Coughing after you eat or after lying down | 0 | 1 | 2 | 3 | 4 | 5 |
| Breathing difficulties or choking episodes | 0 | 1 | 2 | 3 | 4 | 5 |
| Troublesome or annoying cough | 0 | 1 | 2 | 3 | 4 | 5 |
| Sensation of a lump in your throat | 0 | 1 | 2 | 3 | 4 | 5 |
| Heartburn, chest pain, indigestion, acid coming up | 0 | 1 | 2 | 3 | 4 | 5 |

*Reference:* Belafsky PC, Postma GN, Koufman JA. Validity and reliability of the reflux symptom index (RSI). Journal of Voice 16:274-277, 2002.

drainage—that is, too much mucus or phlegm—causing chronic throat clearing. If you have any of those symptoms, especially if you smoke, you should ask your doctor about LPR.

The specialists who most often diagnose and treat people with LPR are ENT (ear, nose, and throat) doctors, also called *otolaryngologists.* The two ENT authors use the *Reflux Symptom Index* (RSI) as a tool for screening patients. You can figure out your own RSI by answering the questions above.

Generally, the magic number for LPR is 15, but the RSI isn't a surefire way to know if you have LPR, because some people with LPR have low RSIs. On the other hand, most people who have LPR have more than one symptom. The average RSI score for a patient coming for treatment in Dr. Koufman's practice is over 20. If you think that you have reflux disease of any kind, go see your doctor.

## REFLUX-RELATED SYMPTOMS AND CONDITIONS (LPR & GERD)

### SYMPTOMS

Heartburn

Regurgitation

Chest pain

Shortness of breath

Choking episodes

Hoarseness

Vocal fatigue

Voice breaks

Chronic throat clearing

Excessive throat mucus

Postnasal drip

Chronic cough

Dysphagia

Difficulty swallowing

Difficulty breathing

Choking episodes

Globus

Food getting stuck

A sensation of a lump in the throat

Intermittent airway obstruction

Chronic airway obstruction

Wheezing

### CONDITIONS

Esophagitis

Dental caries and erosions

Esophageal spasm

Esophageal stricture

Esophageal cancer

Reflux laryngitis

Larynx (laryngeal) cancer

Endotracheal intubation injury

Contact ulcers and granulomas

Posterior glottis stenosis

Arytenoid fixation

Paroxysmal laryngospasm

Globus pharyngeus

Throat cancer

Vocal cord dysfunction

Paradoxical vocal fold movement

Vocal nodules and polyps

Pachydermia laryngis

Recurrent leukoplakia

Polypoid degeneration

Laryngomalacia

Sudden Infant Death Syndrome

Sinusitis and allergic symptoms

Sleep apnea

Asthma

## Red Flags for Reflux

Here are some warning signs and symptoms of serious reflux (both LPR and GERD). Some of these symptoms might indicate the presence of more dangerous conditions as well.

1. Crushing chest pain after eating that makes you wonder if you're having a heart attack; obviously, you should go to an emergency room right away, just in case.
2. Waking in the middle of the night from a sound sleep coughing and gulping air like a fish out of water; this is called laryngospasm. You can't die from it, but it can feel that way.
3. Chronic cough for more than three months with a normal chest x-ray. Reflux is the most common cause of difficult-to-diagnose chronic cough cases.
4. A sensation of a lump in the throat that is there almost all the time, *except* when you are actually eating; usually LPR.
5. Morning hoarseness, progressive (worsening) hoarseness, and painful swallowing can be symptoms of LPR, or even possibly throat cancer. You should see an ENT doctor.

## Reflux and Sleep Disorders

What you eat, how much you eat, and when during the day you eat can all seriously affect the quality of your sleep—which in turn affects your concentration, mood, work habits, and your overall quality of life.

**Avoid overeating and especially overdrinking if you have reflux.** Also, you should never lie down within three hours after a meal, and if you suffer from nighttime reflux, your bed should have a wedge or somehow be elevated to support both your head and your chest. Regular pillows won't help if they only support your head. Elevating the chest makes it more difficult for your dinner to go a-wandering while you sleep; gravity helps.

**Alcohol is trouble for a refluxer at bedtime.** It loosens the valves of the esophagus, allowing stomach contents to reflux. Also, if you go to sleep without a completely clear head, you are officially drunk and may wake up three to four hours later, perspiring and thinking a million different thoughts at once; that's the sign of alcohol withdrawal. Never go to sleep without a clear head. Do breathing exercises, stay awake as long as possible, and drink a lot of water.

**If you wake up coughing in the middle of the night,** there are two likely causes. One is reflux, and the other can be made worse by reflux—sleep apnea, a collapse of your throat, especially during the deeper sleep cycles. Sleep apnea is associated with snoring, but snoring can be caused by reflux as well as other conditions such as being overweight and having chronic congestion of the nasal passages. Sleep apnea is very common and underdiagnosed.

**If you want to get a good night's sleep, eat a light dinner and finish it at least three hours before going to bed.** Avoid salty foods that could cause you to wake dehydrated, and avoid having more than one glass of wine or the equivalent. And, of course, no caffeinated beverages. To really ease into a good night's sleep, try a warm bath, soothing music, and chamomile tea. (Not peppermint!) For more information on how to get a good night's rest, go to Dr. Jordan Stern's website, www.bluesleep.com. It is important to reiterate that late eating is a crucial risk factor for reflux. If we could, we would insist that everyone with reflux close the kitchen by 8:00 p.m., especially people with breathing problems, e.g., asthma. No nightcaps or bedtime snacks—ever!

### From the Case Files of Dr. Koufman

*Felicia was a slender, athletic 70-year-old, a former dancer who kept in shape with an hour of yoga daily. She came seeking help for a chronic cough and morning hoarseness.*

*Her larynx was a disaster. She wasn't responding to medication. That's when she told me about her "healthy" daily regimen: A big evening meal, followed by an hour of yoga, followed by a Granny Smith apple just before bed. Well, here's the thing: You should never exercise on a full stomach or eat within three hours of lying down! Red apples are fine, but for refluxers, a tart (very acidic) Granny Smith apple is like a reflux magnet, especially when it's right before bed.*

*I gave it to Felicia straight. She moved her "big" meal of the day to the afternoon, moved her yoga practice and snacking to earlier time slots, and substituted red for green in her apple-a-day habit. These changes alone were enough to make Felicia completely symptom-free.*

# Maintaining Health: The Reflux Cure

Ear, nose, and throat doctors—including the authors—have listened to their colleagues in gastroenterology (GI) tell them for years that *gastroesophageal reflux disease* (GERD) is a chronic condition often requiring lifelong treatment, and that GERD patients almost always have heartburn and esophagitis (erosions and ulcerations of the swallowing tube between the throat and the stomach). They said the only way to make the diagnosis was by esophageal endoscopy. We believed them.

That is, we believed them until we figured out that many of our patients were *atypical*—they didn't follow the usual progression of what was known as GERD.

Here's an illustrative case example from Dr. Koufman's practice:

About ten years ago, Brad, a high-profile patient from Washington, D.C., wasn't doing well on "maximum antireflux therapy." He had been taking two Prilosec a day and a Zantac before bed. He was reasonable about his diet and avoided late-night snacking. Nevertheless, Brad was still experiencing hoarseness and inflammation of the vocal cords.

One time when Dr. Koufman was visiting him in his office overlooking the Potomac, she noticed that Brad kept sipping a dark brown liquid from a large glass filled with ice. After a few minutes, he went to a small refrigerator and got himself another can of what turned out to be diet cola. Right there was Brad's reflux Achilles' heel.

"You sure do drink a lot of that," remarked Dr. Koufman. "Do you think you have more than a six-pack a day?"

"Oh, magnitudes more," he responded cheerily.

It turned out that Brad drank diet soda all day, every day, which added up to more than a hundred cans a week. His favorite brand scored a very acidic pH 2.9.

Not surprisingly, Brad's reflux laryngitis settled down after he quit the diet soda habit. His symptoms stayed under control until two years later, when he was back in Dr. Koufman's office with a resurgence of his old symptoms. The culprit this time was his latest beverage of choice: a bottled diet lemon iced tea, pH 3.3. Tests of the pH in his larynx and esophagus showed that right after drinking the lemon iced tea, he would reflux for half an hour. Since he drank it all day, the reflux never stopped.

The tea was causing trouble going down and coming up. Once again, Brad's symptoms abated once he stopped his addiction to a harmless-seeming drink.

Carbonated beverages, especially caffeinated soda, are among the most common cause of patients' failure to respond to medical antireflux treatment. But as Brad's case demonstrates, even beverages without bubbles can spell trouble below a certain pH.

We should emphasize that colas are among the worst possible beverages for a refluxer. For one thing, the carbonation increases pressure in the stomach, predisposing you to reflux. For another, caffeine and other chemicals in cola cause the lower esophageal valve to relax, permitting reflux. Finally, the acidic low pH activates the destructive effect of tissue-bound pepsin. For more on pepsin, see the chapters "What You Eat Could Be Eating You" (page 21) and "Reflux Science You Can Digest" (page 159).

## What Else Shouldn't You Drink?

Citrus fruits and juices are very acidic. Alcohol also causes the esophageal valves to relax and cause reflux at night. Beer and white wine are particularly bad for reflux.

The best things for a refluxer to drink? Water! Certain mild herbal teas are fine (such as chamomile), along with nonacidic smoothies, or low-fat and lactose-free milk.

The challenge of defining a "healthy diet" is that there is so much conflicting information available today, especially on the Internet. Some people, for example, say that drinking acidic apple vinegar is good for reflux because it causes the lower esophageal sphincter to tighten up. Unfortunately, this does not appear to be effective, and we believe that it is particularly counterproductive for patients with throat reflux (silent reflux).

From clinical experience, we know that the diet problems of our reflux patients extend beyond the issue of acid. We have long known that high-fat diets are bad for the heart, blood pressure, circulation, bowels, and digestion, and

### From the Case Files of Dr. Koufman

*A 35-year-old venture capitalist had a lifestyle he loved: He didn't eat anything all day so he could save up his calories for night, then he would go out for big, boozy dinners with current and prospective clients. After that, he staggered home late and plopped into bed, only to wake up each morning with a sore throat and do it all over again. He was already on all the available medical treatments, but they didn't make a dent in his symptoms.*

*"Nothing will work until you stop living this crazy way," I told him.*

*"You don't understand," he argued. "It's part of my job."*

*I pointed out that a lot of people do business this way, but that it's not the only way. "You have a choice," I told him. "Change your lifestyle or suffer the consequences."*

*I battled with this man for six months until he finally agreed to go on* ***The Reflux Diet.*** *Guess what? He managed to get well and still be successful in business.*

cause reflux. Fried foods are the worst. The reflux diet is a logical extension of a heart-healthy diet designed to restrict saturated fats.

## Can a Healthy Diet Really Cure Reflux?

About a third of reflux patients just have poor esophageal function and may need medical or surgical treatment. Another third experience relief from symptoms after trying **The Reflux Diet** along with medical treatment. *The final third of our patients find they can achieve complete control over all symptoms just by using the diet alone.*

Especially for those with silent reflux, diet and lifestyle factors strongly influence reflux symptoms one way or the other. You see, reflux is a vicious cycle. The more you have it, the weaker the esophageal valves get. Conversely, diet and lifestyle improvements can reduce symptoms and strengthen the body's defenses against them.

**The Reflux Diet** is essential for the control of disease. It is also essential for healthy self-maintenance. In this book, we offer information that you can use to improve your digestive health overall.

We have extensive clinical experience with **The Reflux Diet.** Many patients who didn't respond to medical treatment improved once they started on it. Usually we recommend a stricter diet for the first two weeks in order to trigger "pepsin wash-out" as a kind of reflux detox. This induction period, during which you consume nothing below pH 5, is followed by a more sustainable and less restricted low-acid diet. Most of the patients following this program notice a big difference in their condition, and, using medical measuring devices, so do we.

Despite overwhelming clinical evidence, almost no long-term dietary studies have looked at acidity as a factor in reflux management. Dr. Koufman reported that 95 percent of her patients improved their symptoms on **The Induction Reflux Diet.** Critics will argue that we have not done long-term controlled studies and therefore have not proven our case against dietary acidity. That is true. However, we believe that the data are too strong to make our patients wait to get relief.

To our knowledge, we are the first physicians to recommend a low-acid diet for reflux patients, and we have basic science to back us up. We also have happy, healthy patients. Additional evidence will come with time, and when it does, some very serious diseases will perhaps be handled quite differently.

For example, we believe that for patients with Barrett's Esophagus (a form of esophageal precancer attributed to reflux), intense, long-term medical treatment should be combined with a long-term acid-free diet (nothing below pH 6). We have shown that pepsin is found in Barrett's biopsies (see Figure 1-B on page 169), and the best treatment regimen might deactivate it. We also believe there is a major link between reflux and asthma and other lung diseases.

Most healthy eaters don't reflux. Most people can be free of reflux and live longer, fuller lives by sticking to a relatively low-acid diet rich in complex carbohydrates, healthy proteins, and oils. The body you have is the last one you're ever going to get. Let this book help you take good care of it!

## From the Case Files of Dr. Koufman

*A prominent fifty-five-year-old ambassador developed hoarseness in 1990. After a few weeks, he went to see an ENT doctor who diagnosed an irregularity on his right vocal cord. Soon thereafter, the lesion was biopsied, and it turned out to be* dysplasia, *which is a kind of precancer. The patient had smoked lightly for only two years during the Korean War, but otherwise had no risk factors.*

*Unfortunately, a few months later, he developed another dysplasia on the other vocal cord. And over the next few years, he developed recurrent dysplasias seven times. Each lesion was surgically removed only to have a new one pop up a few months later. The doctor wasn't sure how to treat the patient, and so, in consultation with an oncologist, it was elected to give the patient's larynx radiation therapy as if he actually had had invasive cancer.*

*A year after the radiation, the ambassador presented with hoarseness, and his examination showed severe reflux laryngitis. The patient was placed on a strict antireflux diet and Prilosec twice a day. Within six months, the larynx appeared to normalize, but because of the radiation and the previous biopsies, the vocal folds were still somewhat scarred and the voice remained husky. In 1998, the author surgically rebuilt the vocal folds, and the patient's voice was restored.*

*In 2008, the patient, feeling quite well, came off the reflux diet and his medicine on his own and, a year later, he again developed severe hoarseness. In January 2010, he was found to have a superficial left vocal fold cancer. This lesion was completely excised with a laser, and the voice was restored.*

*In the ten years from 1998 to 2008, when the ambassador was on the reflux treatment, his larynx was healthy. When he stopped eating right and stopped taking his reflux medication,* that's *when he developed the cancer. Today, he is back on treatment, and he adheres strictly to* ***The Reflux Diet****; his larynx looks fine, and his voice is terrific! The ambassador fully understands what happened to him, and he is now completely compliant in maintaining a low-fat, low-acid diet. Neither of us expects that he will ever get laryngeal cancer again.*

**Comment:** In the author's experience, recurrent reflux-related vocal cord (laryngeal) dysplasia and cancer in the nonsmoker will stop if the patient's reflux is effectively controlled. For more about the relationship between reflux and laryngeal cancer, see pages 167–170 in the chapter "Reflux Science You Can Digest."

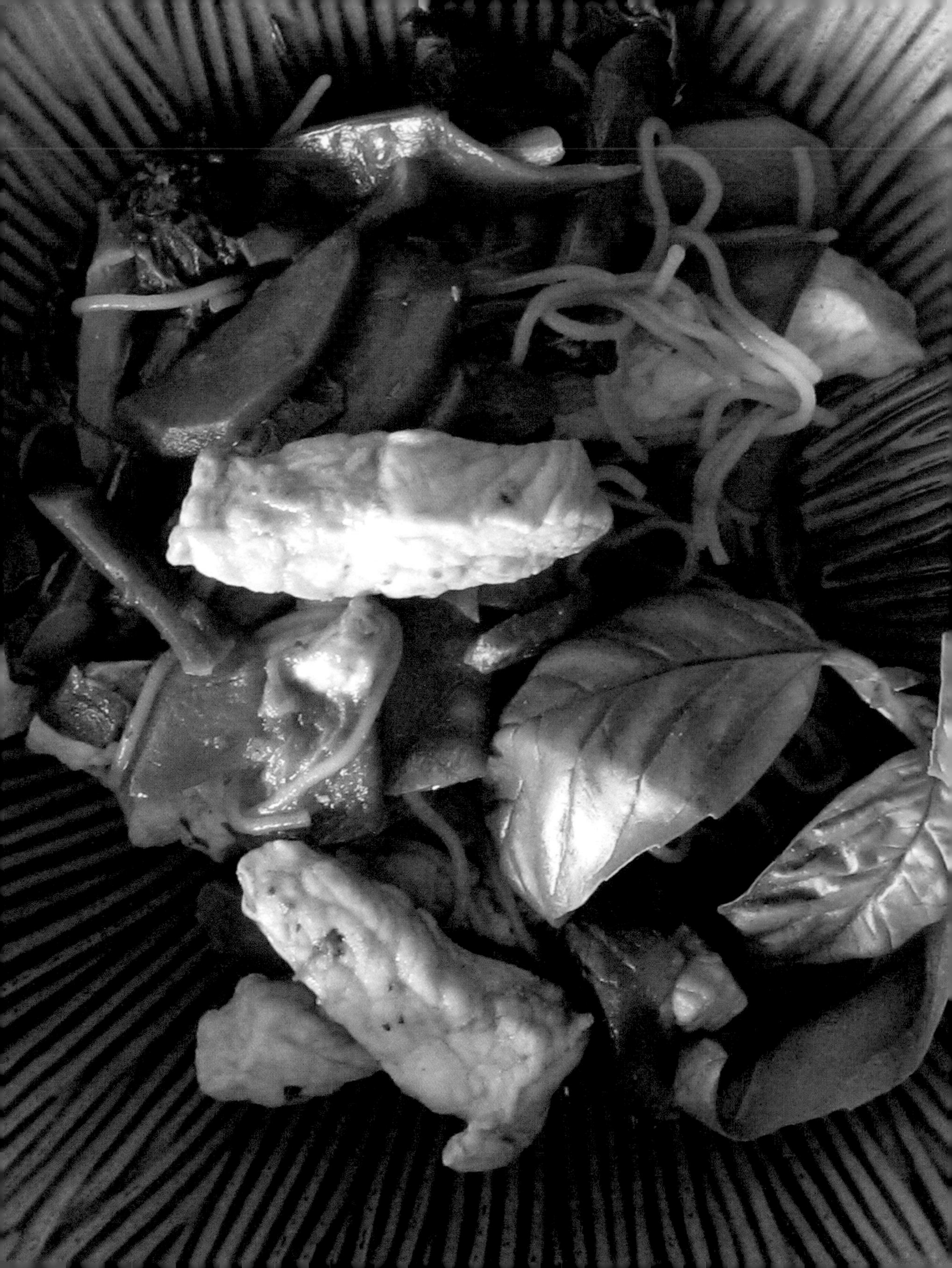

# *the* diet

# Getting Started on the Reflux Diet

If your reflux symptoms are moderate, you can go right to the food lists in subsequent chapters. Just be sure to avoid or limit the foods shown in red in the tables and lists.

If your reflux symptoms are severe, however, you may need to kick things off with two weeks of a strict, acid-free diet, a kind of detox program for your digestive system. It gives your body a respite and deactivates pepsin molecules (those lobsters with their nasty claws) that are still hanging around your throat, esophagus, or elsewhere.

We tried this **Induction Reflux Diet** on some of our patients who weren't responding to typical medical treatments. For two weeks, they ate nothing below pH 5, and they experienced great symptom relief. If your doctor has you on a *proton pump inhibitor* (PPI) such as Nexium, Prilosec, Aciphex, Zegerid, Prevacid, Protonix, omeprazole, or pantoprazole, you should strongly consider this approach.

> **Avoiding acid** means consuming nothing below pH 4. However, if your symptoms are severe, it's well worth considering the even stricter induction phase diet for two weeks, in which you eat nothing below pH 5.

How is the acid-free **Induction Reflux Diet** different from the **Maintenance Reflux Diet?** For one thing, it's strict. During induction, you eat 3–5 meals per day of only the best foods listed below. And no night eating!

Also, the **Induction Reflux Diet** is more limiting. It includes no fruit except for bananas and melons. The main beverage is water—drink at least eight cups of it a day, noncarbonated. (You can still try every recipe in this book, as they are all acceptably low on acid and fat.)

## INDUCTION REFLUX DIET—THE BEST FOODS LIST

([L] means "Limit")

Agave

Avocado

Apple[L] (max. 4 per week, only the reds)

Artificial sweetener[L] (max. 2 tsp per day)

Bagels and (nonfruit) low-fat muffins

Banana (great snack food)

Beans—black, red, lima, lentils, etc.

Bread—whole-grain, rye, unprocessed wheat

Caramel[L] (less than 4 Tbsp/week)

Celery (great snack food)

Chamomile tea—most other herbal teas are not okay

Chicken—grilled/broiled/baked/steamed; no skin

Chicken stock or bouillon

Coffee[L] (one cup per day, best with milk)

Fennel

Fish (including shellfish and sushi)—grilled/broiled/baked/steamed

Ginger—ginger root, powdered or preserved

Green vegetables—excluding green pepper

Herbs—excluding all peppers, citrus, and mustard

Honey

Melon—honeydew, cantaloupe, watermelon

Milk—skim, soy, or Lactaid skim milk recommended

Mushrooms—raw or cooked

Oatmeal and all whole-grain cereals

Olive oil[L] (1–2 Tbsp per day)

Parsley

Pasta—with nonacidic sauce

Pears[L] (max. 4 per week, only if ripe)

Popcorn—plain or salted, no butter

Potatoes—and all of the root vegetables except onions

Red bell peppers[L] (max. 1 per week)

Rice (healthy rice is a staple during induction)
Soups—homemade with noodles and low-acid veggies
Tofu
Turkey breast—organic, no skin
Turnip
Vegetables—raw or cooked, no onion, tomato, peppers
Vinaigrette[L] (1 Tbsp per day)
Water—noncarbonated
Whole-grain breads, crackers, and breakfast cereals

With a little creativity, you can easily sustain the **Induction Reflux Diet.** In brief, the idea is to go two weeks eating only the "Best Foods," and without carbonation, fruit juice, or alcohol.

### From the Case Files of Dr. Koufman

*One of the most dramatic cases I had was a twenty-nine-year-old schoolteacher from Long Island who had all the symptoms of reflux: hoarseness, sore throat, cough, throat clearing, trouble swallowing, etc. She had a horrendous diet. She drank six diet colas a day and loved all the wrong fruits; breakfast for her meant a soda and a grapefruit.*

*The typical treatment for someone like this would be a "proton pump inhibitor" medication and a change in diet, but this young woman was planning to get pregnant and didn't want to be on any meds. Instead, I prescribed the strict* ***Induction Reflux Diet.***

*"But what will I eat?" she wailed.*

*"You'll get up in the morning and have oatmeal," I told her.*

*After two weeks on this diet, the woman's reflux symptom index had gone from 28 (above 15 is bad) down to 4.*

*Not everyone responds this way. We don't expect anyone to get that well that quickly, but the schoolteacher happened to be what we call a "rapid responder." Once she understood and implemented* ***The Reflux Diet****, she was cured.*

# Best Foods for a Refluxer

First and foremost, refer to the **Induction Reflux Diet** "Best Foods" in "Getting Started on the Reflux Diet" (page 45). The foods highlighted below offer plenty of variety and are particularly helpful for reducing reflux. To the degree that you can stick to these, you will be giving yourself the best chance for turning your body into a reflux-free zone.

## Oatmeal

Oatmeal is just about the best breakfast and any-time-of-day snack food we can recommend. It's filling and doesn't cause reflux. Even instant oatmeal with raisins is "legal" because the oatmeal absorbs the acidity of the raisins. (See the recipe for "Oatmeal Marc's Way," page 84.)

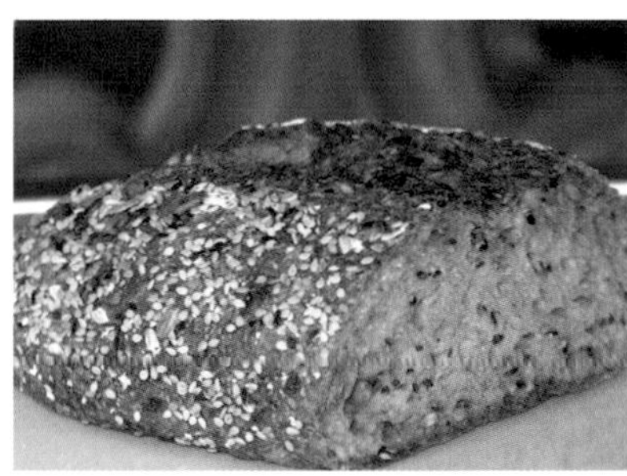

## Whole-Grain Bread

Throughout civilization, bread made from wheat, oats, and barley has been a staple of the human diet. Bread is mentioned in the Bible, but baking didn't catch on until the Middle Ages. Before that, "bread" was more like gruel made from grain. In general, dark bread was considered peasant bread and white bread was considered (literally and figuratively) more refined, but after World War II, refined flour was truly ascendant and whole grains fell out of favor. Only over the last two decades, with our growing concern about the loss of nutrients in refined food products, has whole-grain bread made a comeback.

Whole-grain bread is generally recommended on **The Reflux Diet**, but most of today's wheat has a higher glycemic index (sugar conversion) than the wheat our grandparents ate. Consequently, we suggest limiting bread consumption, especially for our overweight reflux patients, because wheat is converted to sugar and sugar to fat. While whole-grain bread is delicious and makes a good breakfast food, bread should not be consumed with every meal. Replace bread with protein and complex carbohydrates such as lentils, beans, oats, quinoa, and brown rice.

We are now aware that bread (wheat) is a problem for people with gluten sensitivity—celiac disease and gluten ataxia—and for these patients, bread and other wheat-containing foods should be completely eliminated from the diet. We have also identified gluten-sensitive refluxers: a small group whose reflux is triggered by gluten-containing foods. We learned this from patients who reported that a gluten-free diet was key to controlling their reflux. Therefore, we recommend a three-month, gluten-free dietary trial for patients who have recalcitrant reflux, despite an otherwise healthy reflux diet and lifestyle.

In summary, bread is generally a reflux-friendly food, but not for everyone, and **The Reflux Diet** need not be a high-carbohydrate diet with excessive amounts of simple carbs and sugars.

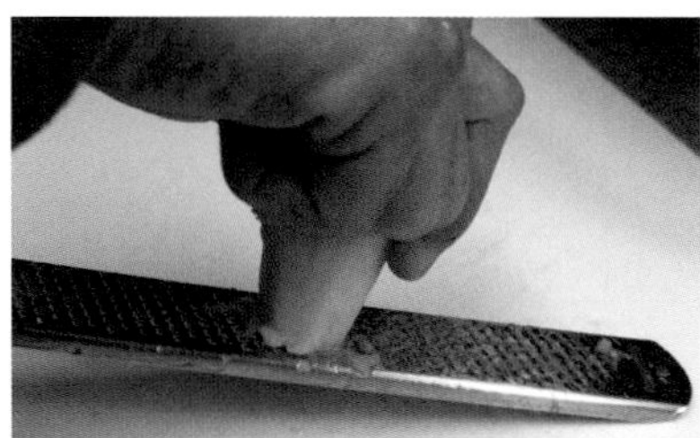

The microplane is one of Chef Marc's favorites. We often use it in our recipes because it's small, easy to work with, versatile, and inexpensive. It works efficiently as a zester and for fine grating and shredding.

## Ginger

In moderation, ginger is one of the best foods for reflux. It's packed with flavor, although it's one of those tastes people either love or hate; it is that distinctive. It has been used throughout history as an anti-inflammatory and as a treatment for gastrointestinal conditions. Our patients routinely give it a thumbs-up, and they aren't unanimous about too many foods.

Ginger root can easily be peeled, sliced, diced, or shaved using a microplane. We use it in this book for cooking and in smoothies.

## Aloe Vera

Aloe vera is famous as a natural healing agent. It also seems to treat reflux. It is available as a living plant, but leaves are sometimes sold separately in groceries and health-food stores. (Avoid aloe bottled beverages.) We use aloe vera in our recipes as a thickener and for congealing liquids. For more information, there is a comprehensive blog post on aloe vera on www.refluxcookbookblog.com.

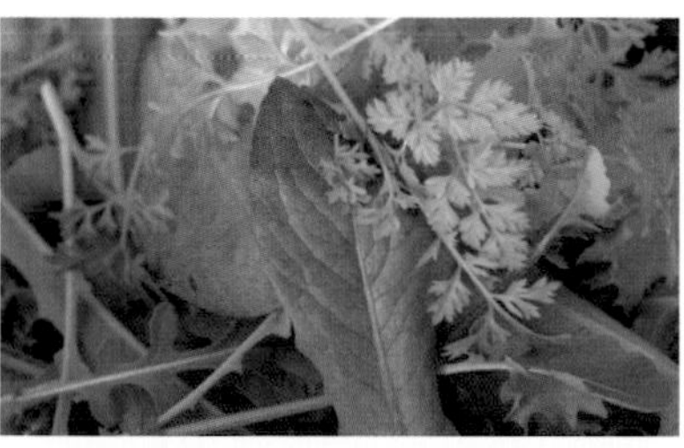

### Salad

You could do worse than to eat a salad every day. Salad is a primary meal for refluxers, although tomatoes and onions should be avoided as well as cheese and high-fat dressings. We allow dressings with some acid or fat, but only one tablespoon (or less)—as measured, not guesstimated!

### Banana

Bananas make a great snack, and at pH 5.6, they're great for reflux. However, about 1 percent of refluxers find their condition is worsened by bananas. That number is so small that we are not listing banana as an idiosyncratic food, but keep in mind that what works for most people may not work for you.

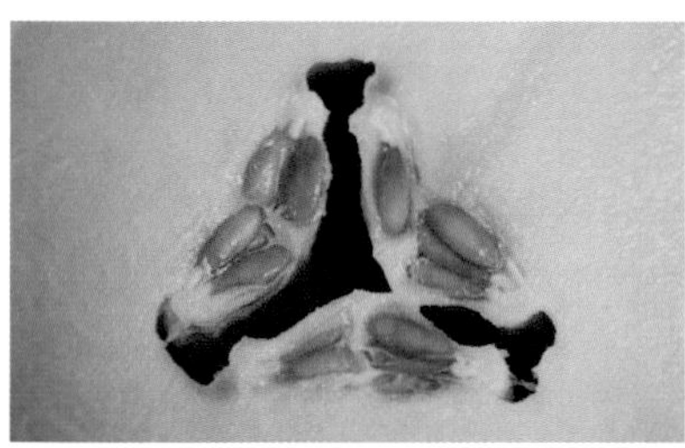

### Melon

Melon (pH 6.1) is good for reflux. However, as with bananas, a small percentage of those with reflux need to avoid it. The number is so small (1–2 percent) that we are not listing melon as an idiosyncratic food. Included in the good-for-reflux category are honeydew, cantaloupe, and watermelon.

### Fennel

Fennel (pH 6.9) is a great food for reflux and actually seems to improve stomach function. This crunchy vegetable has a unique taste, a mild licorice flavor. Sliced thin (the white bottom part), it makes a great salad with arugula and baby spinach. It's also great in chicken dishes, and makes a fine snack if you love the taste.

### Chicken and Turkey

Poultry is a staple of **The Reflux Diet.** It can be boiled, baked, grilled, or sautéed (but not fried!), and you must remove the skin, which is high in fat. (Check out the four poultry recipes under "Entrées.")

### Fish/Seafood

Seafood is another staple of **The Reflux Diet.** It should be baked, grilled, or sautéed, never fried. Shrimp, lobster, and other shellfish are also fine on this diet. We recommend wild fish, not farm raised.

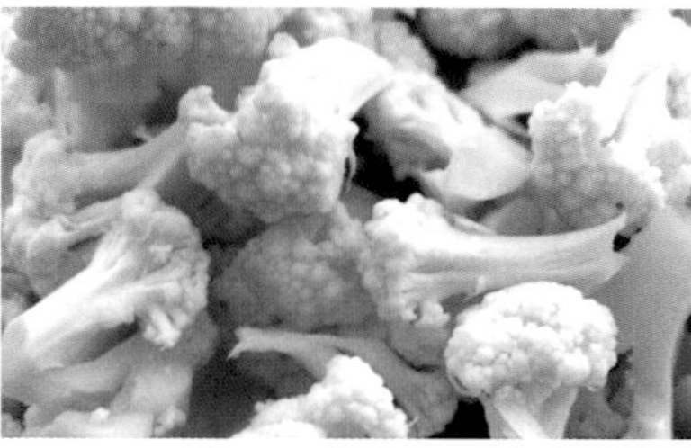

### Cauliflower, Broccoli, Asparagus, Green Beans, and Other Greens

These are all great foods for the refluxer. Pretty much all of the green and the root vegetables are good.

### Celery

Celery has almost no calories because of its high water content. It is also an excellent source of roughage and an appetite suppressant.

### Parsley

For thousands of years, parsley has been used as a medicinal herb to settle the stomach and aid digestion. Flat-leaf and curly parsley are widely available, and they make a great seasoning and garnish.

### Couscous and Rice

Couscous (semolina wheat), bulgur wheat, and rice (especially brown rice) are all outstanding foods for reflux. As we like to say, a complex carbohydrate is a good carbohydrate.

## Are Salt and Pepper Okay?

**Salt does not cause reflux**, and **The Reflux Diet** is not a salt-restricted diet. We use salt and items like capers in some of our recipes. For those with no personal or family history of hypertension (high blood pressure), it appears that the salt they consume is simply excreted without causing problems. If your doctor has put you on a salt restriction, however, you must adjust recipes accordingly.

As for pepper, even in small amounts it's one of those pesky, unpredictable, idiosyncratic foods. For some people, pepper sets off their reflux. We think small ("pinch") amounts of black pepper added in cooking are fine, but you probably need to limit your use of cracked black, white, or red peppers that are added after cooking to a finished dish.

People with reflux-related chronic cough should avoid pepper (especially cayenne). The same goes for hot peppers and hot pepper sauce.

## Should I Buy Organic Food?

We generally recommend organic food on principle, and we especially insist on organic poultry and fish.

Organic free-range chickens are leaner and a little less tender, but they more than make up for this in taste. It's interesting to note that it takes several months to raise an organic chicken in the wild, while commercial, coop-restricted, farm-raised chickens take only a month.

Fish is also an important part of **The Reflux Diet.** We suggest having fresh fish at least twice a week.

Finally, the best whole-grain breads are organic, so seek them out at farmer's markets and health-food stores.

### From the Case Files of Dr. Koufman

*One of the top touring rock stars in the world came to see me when he was performing in New York. He was worried because his voice was frequently raspy and he had a full slate of performances scheduled.*

*He was into raw foods and always traveled with a personal chef. Sounds healthy, right? But his raw foods included tons of citrus fruit. I put him on an acid-free diet and explained the rules to his chef.*

*This was before we had tested as many foods in the lab as we have now, so we weren't sure about certain items. For weeks, I received a barrage of anxious e-mails from the rock star's chef. "What about tofu?" "How's corn on the cob?" Tofu is fine. Corn is fine. Some of the foods he was into were new to me.*

*It took a while, but the chef sorted things out and developed a menu that worked for the star and brought him relief. Now, his voice is fine.*

# Notoriously Bad Reflux Foods

Some foods are almost universally problematic for people with reflux. The best strategy for the refluxer is to avoid the "bad" foods. Our list of foods to avoid is based on the medical literature and our experience treating thousands of patients. The worst offenders always seem to be alcohol, chocolate, and carbonated beverages (especially acidic ones with caffeine).

## Foods That Are Notorious For Causing Reflux (Red is Bad)

Chocolate (especially high-fat milk chocolate)
Soda (all carbonated beverages)
Alcohol (beer, liquor, and wine)
Any deep-fried food
Bacon, sausage, ribs
Cream sauce (e.g., Alfredo)
Fatty meat (e.g., high-fat hamburgers)
Butter, margarine, lard, shortening
Coffee, tea (caffeinated beverages)
Mint (especially peppermint and spearmint)
High-fat nuts (peanut butter)
Hot sauces and pepper
Citrus fruit/juices

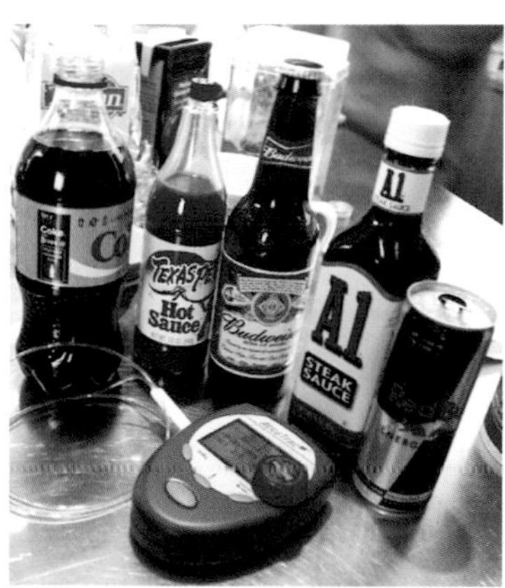

SAY GOODBYE TO THESE

These are way bad! Unfortunately, these foods constitute over half of many people's diet. Some of these foods are so common they warrant further explanation:

### Chocolate

Bad news for chocolate lovers: chocolate seems to cause more reflux than any other food. It's a triple whammy: (1) Chocolate contains caffeine and other stimulants such as theobromine, both of which cause reflux; (2) Chocolate is high in fat, and fat causes reflux; and (3) Chocolate is also high in cocoa, and cocoa causes reflux. Theoretically, dark chocolate isn't as bad as high-fat milk chocolate, but let's face it: All chocolate is bad for reflux.

### Soda (all carbonated beverages)

Some people drink more than a six-pack of soda a day, yet this is one of the biggest causes of reflux. The bubbles of carbonation expand inside the stomach, and the increased pressure contributes to reflux. In addition, sodas with caffeine and those that are very acidic (below pH 4) are worse. Of the beverages we tested, Coke, Tab, and Diet Pepsi were the most acidic. By the way, pH 4 and below is within the normal range for stomach acid! All carbonation is suspect, so we recommend abstinence. Please quit!

### Fried Food

*Fried food is the single most recognized cause of reflux.* It is also the food most associated with heartburn, which is chest pain from esophageal reflux. Deep fried (even not so deep fried) foods are on the bad list because of their high fat content.

> **Sorry to break the bad news,** but there are things all refluxers must give up for sure: chocolate, soda pop, fried food, and late-night eating.

### Alcohol

Beer, liquor, and wine are believed to contribute to reflux. We didn't test the pH of too many alcoholic beverages, and the ones we did test are not very acidic. However, alcohol is believed to relax the valve at the bottom of the esophagus (where it joins the stomach), leading to reflux. Abstain if you can; otherwise, indulge in moderation, and completely avoid acidic mixers like cranberry and orange juice or soda.

### ACIDITY (pH) OF SOME POPULAR CARBONATED BEVERAGES

|  |  |
|---|---|
| Coca-Cola | 2.8 |
| Tab—diet | 2.9 |
| Pepsi—diet | 2.9 |
| Mountain Dew—diet | 3.1 |
| Prosecco (Mionetto) | 3.1 |
| Ginger ale (Seagram's) | 3.2 |
| Coke Zero | 3.3 |
| Pepsi | 3.5 |
| Sprite Zero—diet | 3.7 |
| Coca-Cola—diet | 3.7 |
| Seltzer (Seagram's original) | 3.8 |
| Red Bull—energy drink | 3.9 |
| Sparkling water (Poland Spring) | 4.3 |
| Cream soda—diet (Dr. Brown's) | 4.5 |

### Cream/Butter (high-fat dairy products)

*All high-fat foods cause reflux.* There is no reason to believe that one high-fat butter or cheese is better than another in this regard. If you have reflux and a serious cheese habit, something has to give. Here's the negotiating point: We'll let you use a small amount of these foods as flavorings, but not as main ingredients. *We believe in low fat, not no fat.*

### Beef and Other High-fat Meats

It's about the fat content. In general, fatty cuts of beef stay longer in the stomach. We recommend a lean cut of beef only once a week.

### Caffeine

One cup of coffee or espresso a day is fine, but people who drink coffee all day long are courting reflux if they don't have it already. We recommend switching to herbal teas such as chamomile. Green tea is okay if lightly brewed.

### Hot Sauce and Hot Peppers

Forget it; these cause problems. *Avoid.*

### Mints

Mints cause reflux, especially spearmint and peppermint. *Avoid.*

## Idiosyncratic (Usually Bad) Foods

Watch out for *idiosyncratic* foods. For many people with reflux, there are certain foods that make their reflux worse even though others can eat them with no ill effects. Idiosyncratic foods are the "maybe bad for reflux" or "often-bad" foods. Below is a list of the most common ones. We generally do not use these foods in our recipes unless they are present in small amounts and/or combined with certain ingredients that make the pH of the dish acceptable.

### From the Case Files of Dr. Koufman

*A woman who ran a language school in Moscow came to me after seeing two gastroenterologists, one in Russia and one in New York. Both of them performed an endoscopy and told her they saw no signs of reflux, but that didn't explain why she was still suffering from chronic hoarseness, throat clearing, and a cough.*

*I quickly discerned that she had silent reflux, and I asked about her diet. It turned out she was addicted to the two things that are responsible for more reflux in my patients than anything else: chocolate and soda pop.*

*Chocoholics and soda-pop fiends hate to give up those addictions, but the woman from Russia said she would do whatever it took. I knew she had been successful even before our next appointment, because suddenly I was getting a lot of new patients from Russia. The woman had been so happy with her results that she was sharing the news in all the online Russian chat rooms.*

## Most Common Idiosyncratic (Usually Bad) Reflux Foods

Tomatoes

Garlic

Onion

Nuts

Apples

Cucumber

Green peppers

Spicy food

Some herbal teas (chamomile is the best tea for refluxers)

Coffee

### From the Case Files of Dr. Koufman

*Melissa's problem all came down to macadamia nuts. This slender, fifty-eight-year-old editor from Chicago came to see me because of a chronic cough. She was already taking medication, but had failed to respond to it.*

*A laryngeal examination showed that Melissa had reflux, but the big problem wasn't in her larynx; it was in her pantry. Macadamia nuts were a trigger food for her—the one food she couldn't resist—and she ate them by the bagful.*

*As soon as we identified the chief culprit, Melissa changed her snacking habits, and her cough subsided.*

Unfortunately, a few people with reflux sometimes have problems with even the "Good-for-Reflux" foods. One of the challenges of managing reflux is that almost everything is bad for someone. We think banana is a good food for most refluxers, but a tiny percentage suffer more with bananas. If you know or suspect that a particular food causes you problems—even if it is on our "good list"—then avoid it.

# Avoiding Acidic Foods and Beverages

By reading the previous chapters of this book, you hopefully understand that reflux disease is caused by both acid and pepsin, and that most of the inflammation and tissue damage is due to pepsin—remember those lobsters? When you have pepsin on or in the lining membranes of your throat, esophagus, etc., it doesn't take a lot of acid to activate it. That's why we recommend a low-acid diet.

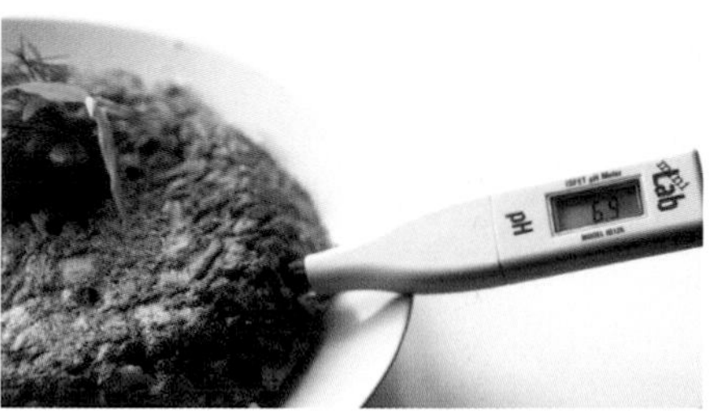


We tested the pH (acidity) of many foods and beverages. For the reflux diet, foods and beverages below pH 4 are too acidic. For the first two weeks of the diet, we recommend avoiding anything pH 5 and lower. Remember, low pH means high acidity, and the best pH values for foods/beverages are pH 5–7. After the initial two weeks, pH 4–5 foods are okay.

If you have severe reflux and/or your doctor has prescribed special antireflux medication, you should consider the **Induction Reflux Diet** for two to four weeks—that means eat nothing below pH 5. If your reflux is not severe, then the **Maintenance Reflux Diet** will do; that is, you should restrict your diet to nothing below pH 4. By the way, there is a moderate "middle ground." The listed red items . . . it doesn't mean that you can never have any of these foods or beverages . . . but the red items are bad for reflux. When you are well, by all means, you may have some of those red items some of the time.

Remember, the pH scale is tricky; pH 4 is ten times as acidic as pH 5, and stomach acid is usually between pH 1 and pH 4. In the lists below, red means that the pH is less than 4. Green is greater than pH 4. Also note that some restricted foods and beverages are red because they are bad for reflux for some reason other than just acidity (pH).

## ACIDITY (pH) OF COMMON DRINKS AND BEVERAGES
## AVOID, VERY ACIDIC (LESS THAN PH 4.0)

([B] means "Bad for Reflux" for reasons other than acidity)

| | pH |
|---|---|
| Coca-Cola | 2.8 |
| Pomegranate cranberry juice (Langer's) | 2.8 |
| Tab—diet soda | 2.9 |
| Diet Pepsi | 2.9 |
| Cranberry juice (Tropicana) | 2.9 |
| Gatorade—fruit punch | 3.0 |
| Cognac | 3.0 |
| Mountain Dew—diet | 3.1 |
| Prosecco (Mionetto) | 3.1 |
| Iced tea (Lipton lemon) | 3.2 |
| Ginger ale (Seagram's) | 3.2 |
| Snapple—diet lemon | 3.3 |
| Coke Zero | 3.3 |
| Pepsi | 3.5 |
| Sprite Zero—diet soda | 3.7 |
| Diet Coke | 3.7 |
| Cranberry pomegranate juice (Knudsen) | 3.7 |
| Orange juice | 3.8 |
| Seltzer (Seagram's original) | 3.8 |
| Tomato juice (Campbell's from concentrate) | 3.9 |
| Red Bull—energy drink | 3.9 |
| V8 vegetable juice | 4.2 |
| Sparkling water[B] (Poland Spring) | 4.3 |
| Stolichnaya vodka[B] on the rocks—lemon twist | 4.4 |
| Budweiser beer[B] | 4.5 |
| Cream soda[B] (Dr. Brown's diet) | 4.5 |
| Vodka[B] (Absolut) | 4.7 |
| Pellegrino[B] | 4.8 |
| Coffee (strong black) Limit one cup a day | 5.0 |
| Tea (Chinese white jasmine) Limit one cup a day | 5.6 |
| Coffee (with milk) Limit one cup a day | 6.2 |
| Bottled water—flat (Poland Spring) | 6.9 |
| New York City tap water | 7.0 |
| Milk (Lactaid fat-free) | 7.0 |
| Milk—2% Organic | 7.5 |

**REMEMBER: Red Is Bad and Green Is Good**

## ACIDITY OF FRESH FRUITS, VEGETABLES, AND COMMON FOODS

([B] means "Bad for Reflux" for reasons other than acidity)

| | pH |
|---|---|
| Lime | 2.7 |
| Lemon | 2.9 |
| Pineapple | 3.1 |
| Apples—Macoun | 3.2 |
| Nectarines | 3.3 |
| Pomegranate | 3.3 |
| Grapefruit—pink | 3.4 |
| Kiwi | 3.4 |
| Strawberries | 3.5 |
| Grape—green, seedless | 3.6 |
| Peaches | 3.6 |
| Apples—Granny Smith | 3.6 |
| Pineapple | 3.7 |
| Blackberries | 3.7 |
| Blueberries | 3.7 |
| Mango | 3.7 |
| Apples—McIntosh | 3.7 |
| Orange—navel | 3.8 |
| Cherries | 3.9 |
| Apples—Fuji | 4.0 |
| Yogurt—1% peach | 4.0 |
| Apples—Red Delicious | 4.2 |
| Apples—Gala | 4.2 |
| Raspberries | 4.2 |
| Yogurt—1% milk fat plain | 4.3 |
| Tomatoes[B]—Mexican | 4.3 |
| Tomatoes[B]—Roma (raw or cooked) | 4.4 |
| Tomatoes[B]—Beefsteak (cooked) | 4.5 |
| Tomatoes[B]—Mexican (cooked) | 4.8 |
| Bell pepper—orange | 4.8 |
| Bell pepper—red | 4.9 |
| Bell pepper—Italian stuffing pepper | 5.0 |
| Bell pepper—green | 5.1 |
| Pear—Bosc | 5.3 |
| Gherkin | 5.4 |

| | pH |
|---|---|
| Banana | 5.6 |
| Potato—Idaho | 5.7 |
| Squash—acorn | 5.9 |
| Potato—Yukon gold | 6.0 |
| Cucumber | 6.0 |
| Endive | 6.0 |
| Onion[B]—white | 6.0 |
| Eggplant | 6.0 |
| Cabbage—green | 6.0 |
| Cabbage—Savoy | 6.1 |
| Melon—ripe cantaloupe | 6.1 |
| Mushrooms—domestic | 6.1 |
| Yams | 6.1 |
| Radish—red or black | 6.1 |
| Beets—red | 6.1 |
| Parsley—Italian flat leaf | 6.1 |
| Squash—spaghetti | 6.2 |
| Green beans—raw | 6.2 |
| Green beans—cooked | 6.3 |
| Cabbage—red | 6.3 |
| Turnip | 6.2 |
| Broccoli—cooked | 6.2 |
| Broccoli—raw | 6.3 |
| Onion[B]—Spanish, yellow, raw | 6.3 |
| Onion[B]—white, sautéed | 6.4 |
| Ginger | 6.5 |
| Mushroom—portobello | 6.5 |
| Parsnip | 6.6 |
| Zucchini | 6.6 |
| Pancake batter—banana/oatmeal | 6.8 |
| Corn | 6.9 |
| Fennel | 6.9 |
| Carrots | 7.0 |
| Oatmeal with 2% milk | 7.2 |
| Avocado | 7.8 |

**REMEMBER:** Red Is Bad and Green Is Good

## ACIDITY OF COMMON PREPARED FOODS, DRESSINGS, AND CONDIMENTS

Prepared foods are more acidic than fresh
because of preservatives added to extend shelf life.

| | pH |
|---|---|
| Hot sauce (Texas Pete) | 3.1 |
| Mandarin oranges (Dole) | 3.2 |
| Mustard—yellow (White Rose) | 3.2 |
| Applesauce (Mott's original) | 3.4 |
| Barbecue sauce (Kraft original) | 3.4 |
| Ketchup (Heinz) | 3.4 |
| Mango (Del Monte "Sunfresh mango in syrup") | 3.4 |
| Worcestershire Sauce (Lea & Perrins) | 3.4 |
| Caesar dressing (Newman's Own) | 3.5 |
| Mustard—Dijon (Grey Poupon) | 3.6 |
| Thousand Island dressing (Kraft) | 3.6 |
| Barbecue sauce (Bull's-Eye original) | 3.7 |
| Pickle—crunchy, dill (B&G) | 3.7 |
| Salsa—mild, chunky (Tostitos) | 3.7 |
| Russian dressing (Wishbone) | 3.8 |
| Ranch dressing—reduced fat (Kraft) | 3.9 |
| Tomato sauce (Del Monte) | 3.9 |
| Tomato juice (Campbell's from concentrate) | 3.9 |
| Tomatoes—whole, peeled (San Marzano) | 3.9 |
| Tomato paste[B] (Hunt) | 4.0 |
| Tomatoes[B]—diced (San Marzano) | 4.0 |
| Tomato sauce[B]—mushroom (Prego Italian) | 4.0 |
| Tomato sauce[B]—pizza, quick (Ragu) | 4.1 |
| Tomato sauce[B]—organic (Del Monte) | 4.1 |
| Tomatoes[B]—whole, peeled (Best Yet) | 4.1 |
| Salsa[B]—tomato, chipotle (Rosa Mexicano) | 4.1 |
| V8[B] vegetable juice | 4.2 |
| Agave nectar (Sweet Cactus Farms) | 4.5 |
| Yogurt | 4.8 |
| Italian dressing (Zesty Kraft) | 5.2 |
| Green beans—canned, cut (Green Giant) | 5.2 |
| Peas—canned, small (Le Sueur) | 5.8 |
| Corn—whole kernel (Del Monte) | 6.6 |
| Olives—black, pitted (Best Brand) | 7.3 |

# Delicious Low-Fat Cooking

The **Reflux Diet Cookbook & Cure** offers one of the healthiest sustainable diets in the world. It is low in fat, acid, and caffeine, and high in whole grains, root vegetables, fruit, fish, and poultry. Many of the tasty high-fat foods that are usually prohibited on the typical antireflux diet, such as cheese, are used in small amounts as flavorings in our recipes.

## *Low* Fat, Not *No* Fat

There is a misconception about fat in food. Fat brings a pleasurable feeling of richness and enhances the flavor of many dishes. That's why food with absolutely no fat is usually unappealing.

We believe that there's no reason to deprive yourself of the flavor, texture, and satiety factor of fat—as long as you consume a controlled amount of it in a suitable ratio to the amount of food in the entire recipe.

Many sauces in traditional cooking include a lot of butter, crème fraîche, cream, etc., and can end up being 30–90 percent fat. In **The Reflux Diet Cookbook** recipes, we use ingredients that average out at about 10 percent fat content. If you start with these recipes and foods, you can always slightly increase the amount of fatty ingredients to taste.

We use fat in the recipes as a flavoring agent. It is not used in huge amounts. For this reason, we like to use the most flavorful fats, such as extra-virgin olive oil, butter, imported Parmesan, or an extra-sharp cheddar cheese.

Since fat is harmful in great amounts, we choose the strongest in flavor. An egg contains 5 grams of fat, all of it located in the yolk, but the white has no fat content. People with high cholesterol should avoid yolks, but the egg yolk adds a lot of flavor to food, and the amount is so little (less than 10 percent of the whole egg) that we don't mind using it in our recipes.

(Note: For some people with reflux, eggs are an idiosyncratic food.)

## Chef Marc's Favorite Flavorings for Reflux Recipes

Capers

Anchovies

Vinaigrette

Dijon mustard

Toasted sesame seeds

White or red miso paste

Low-sodium soy sauce

Salt (not pepper)

Brown sugar

Lemon or orange zest (peel only)

Maple syrup (D-grade has more flavor)

Cheese—Parmesan, cheddar, Roquefort

Herbs—cilantro, basil, dill, parsley, oregano, rosemary, lemongrass, cardamon, cafir, lime leaves, tarragon

Whole milk or 2%

Dry mushrooms

Nonfat yogurt

Fish sauce

Ginger

## Fatty Foods That Can Be Used in Small Amounts

Butter

Olive oil

Whole egg

Toasted nuts

Salad dressings

Toasted sesame seeds

Citrus oils from zest (orange, lemon, lime)

Italian Parmesan or Romano cheese

Cheddar cheese extra sharp (Vermont or other)

If you simply cannot tolerate one or more of these, then you will have to get along without the corresponding flavors. But for most people with reflux, the above items in small amounts are excellent seasonings and flavorings, and they work well in the recipes in this book. In our recipes, we judiciously limit the ingredients that are high in acid, such as vinegar, citrus, and certain fruits.

Bottled salad dressings, even relatively acidic ones such as vinaigrette, are okay when used sparingly—a tablespoon or less. By tossing the salad, you can get full flavor with a small amount of dressing.

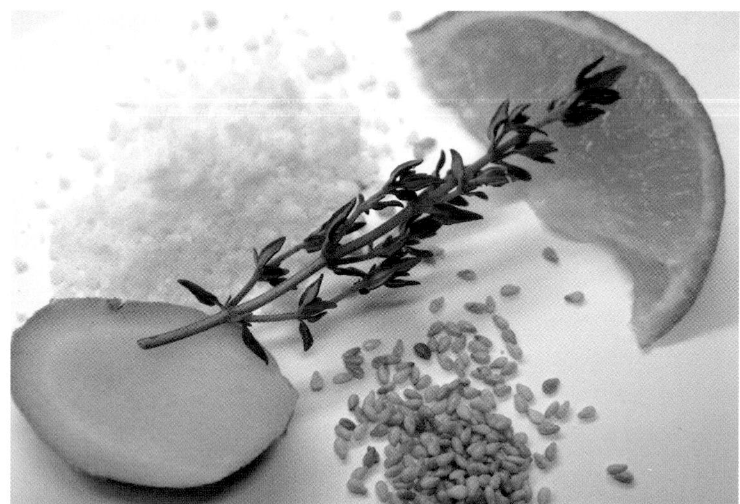

Among Marc's favorite flavorings for cooking are orange zest, toasted sesame seeds, fresh ginger, Parmesan cheese, and fresh herbs.

## Some Notes From Chef Marc About the Recipes in This Book

I like to use stainless steel pots. I avoid aluminum pots as much as possible, because the aluminum tends to react with foods, especially the acidic kind.

My ideal cooking vessel is made of a sandwich of stainless steel with an aluminum core. Aluminum is a good heat conductor, and in a stainless-steel sandwich, it avoids exposure to the food's acidity. These pots can also be washed in the dishwasher. My preferred brand is All-Clad, but there are other great brands offering aluminum-sandwich construction, such as Calphalon.

You'll notice a lot of recipes in this book call for chicken stock. I like the way chicken stock adds a mild, delicious taste, and because the vegetables themselves have been strained out, you won't suffer any of the possible side effects of onion or garlic.

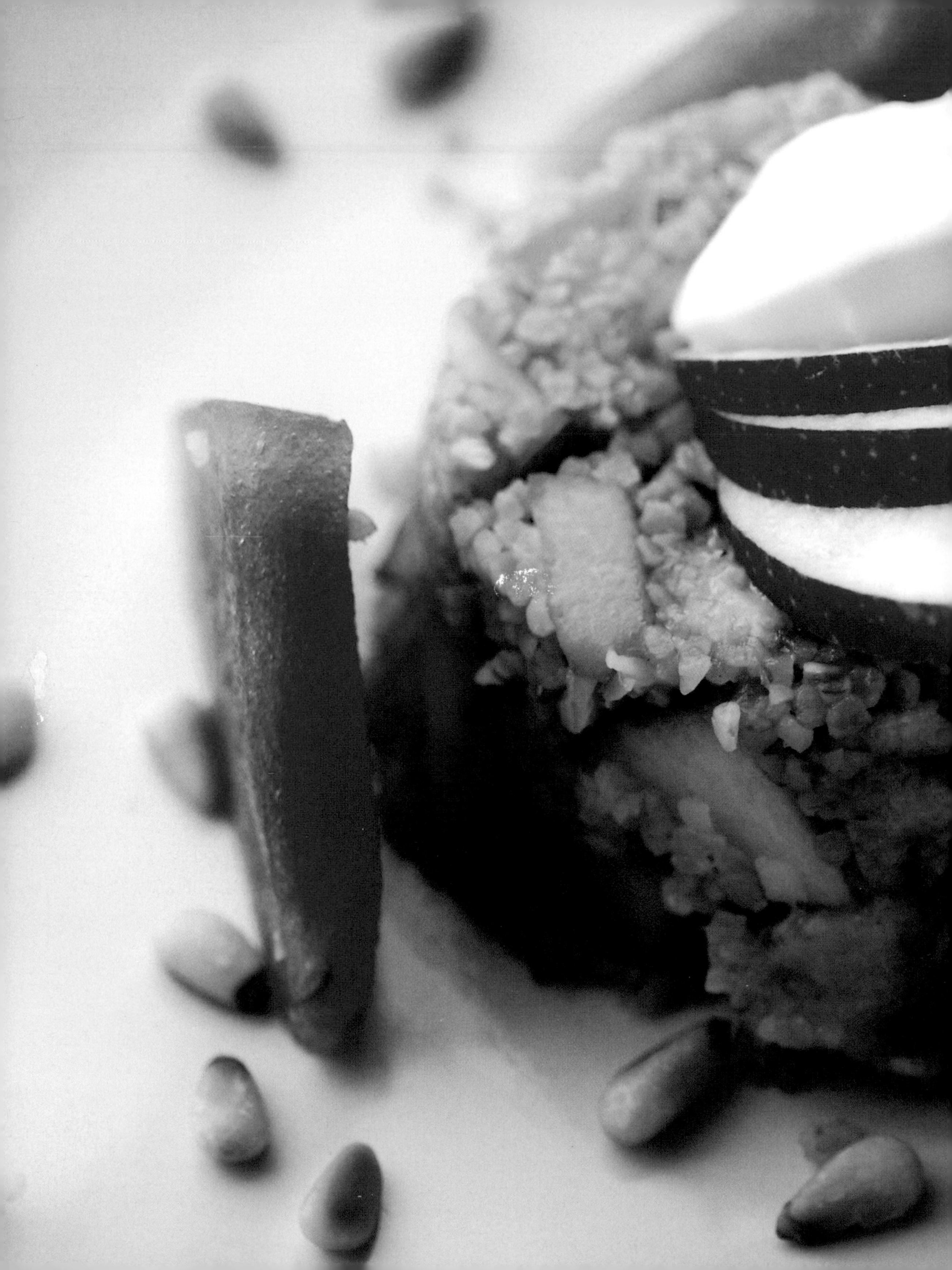

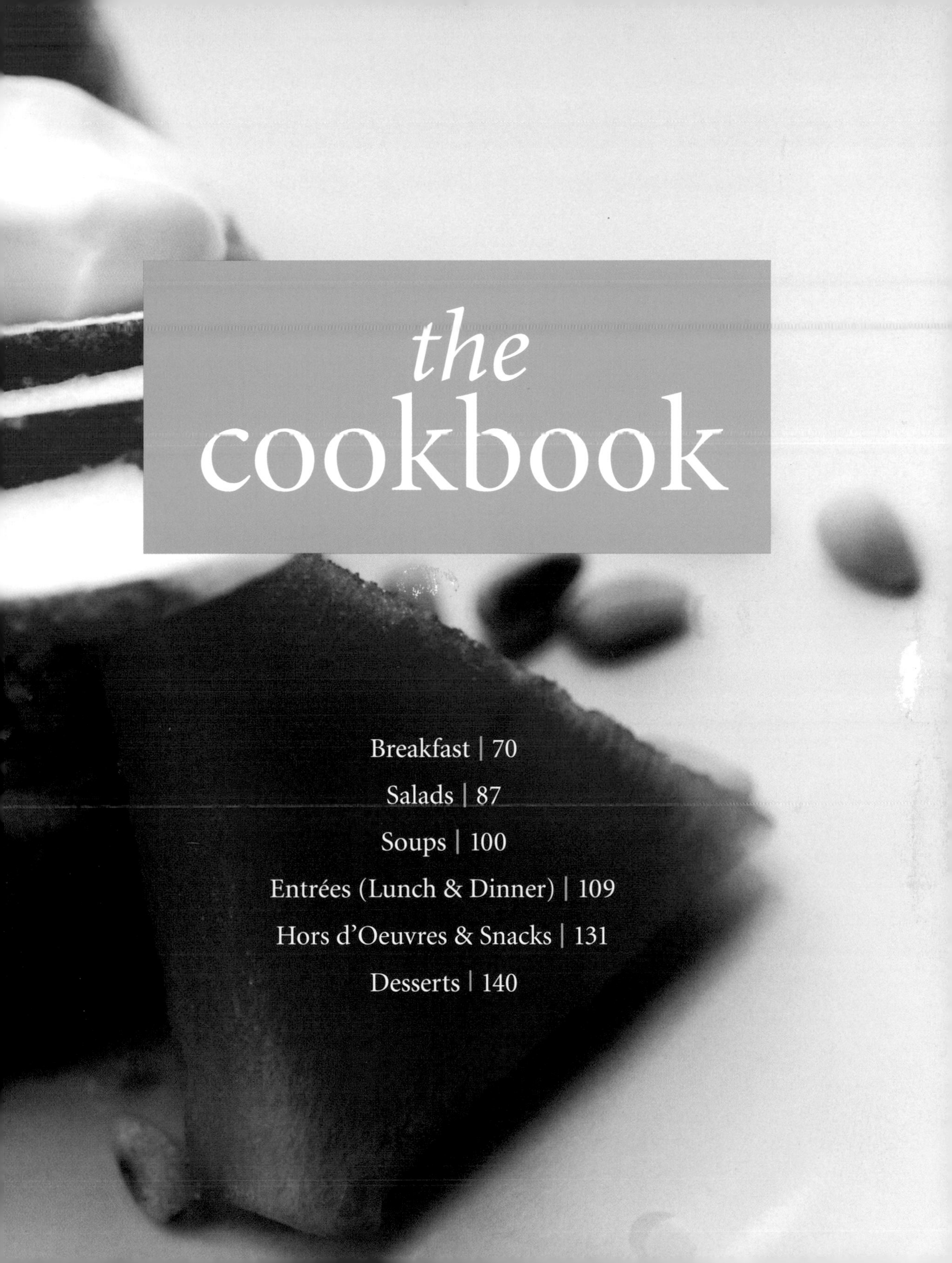

# *the* cookbook

Breakfast | 70

Salads | 87

Soups | 100

Entrées (Lunch & Dinner) | 109

Hors d'Oeuvres & Snacks | 131

Desserts | 140

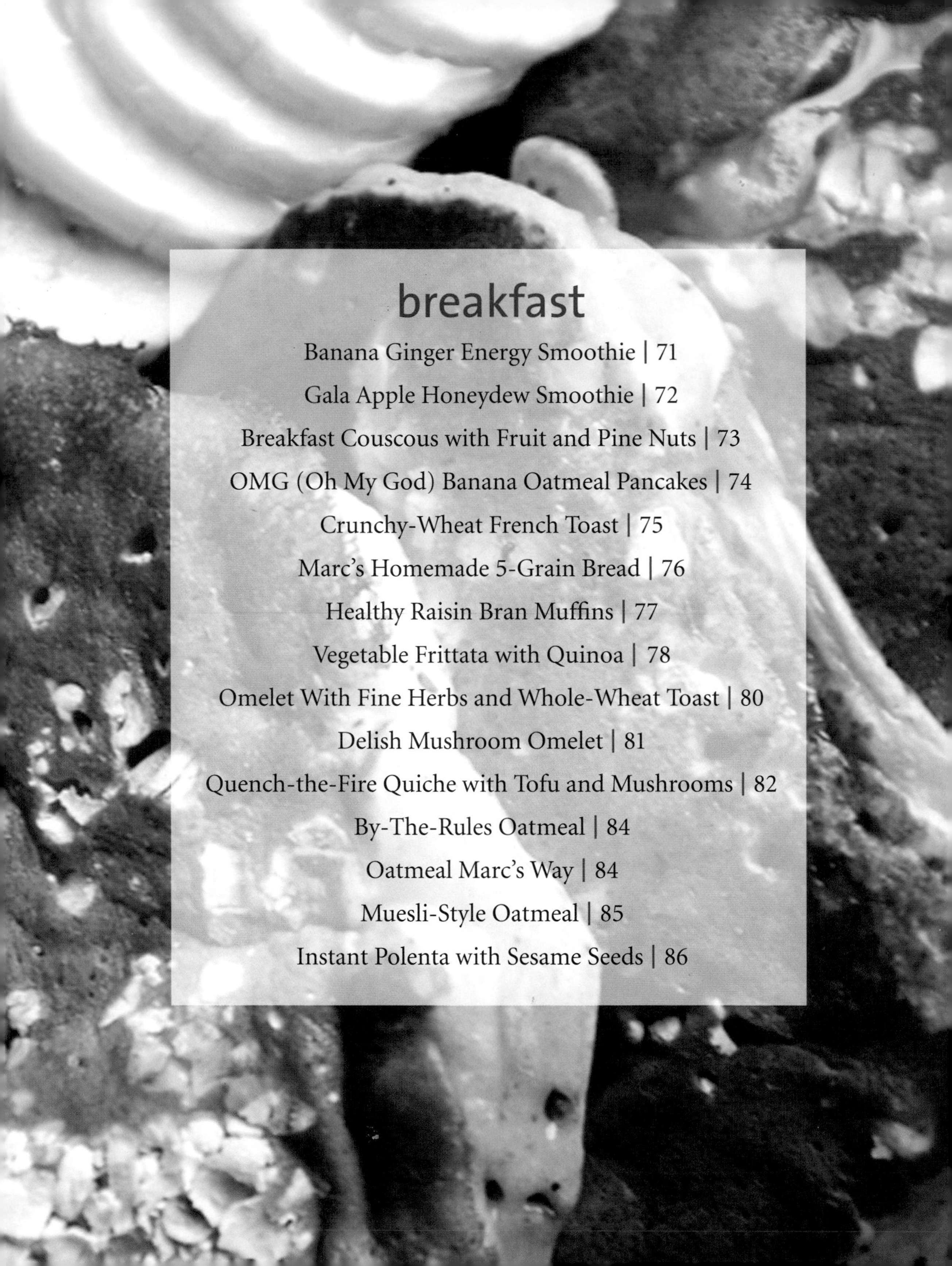

# breakfast

Banana Ginger Energy Smoothie | 71

Gala Apple Honeydew Smoothie | 72

Breakfast Couscous with Fruit and Pine Nuts | 73

OMG (Oh My God) Banana Oatmeal Pancakes | 74

Crunchy-Wheat French Toast | 75

Marc's Homemade 5-Grain Bread | 76

Healthy Raisin Bran Muffins | 77

Vegetable Frittata with Quinoa | 78

Omelet With Fine Herbs and Whole-Wheat Toast | 80

Delish Mushroom Omelet | 81

Quench-the-Fire Quiche with Tofu and Mushrooms | 82

By-The-Rules Oatmeal | 84

Oatmeal Marc's Way | 84

Muesli-Style Oatmeal | 85

Instant Polenta with Sesame Seeds | 86

# Banana Ginger Energy Smoothie

***Serves 3***
***Nutritional information per serving***
Calories 178
Protein 10g
Carbohydrates 33g
Fat 2g

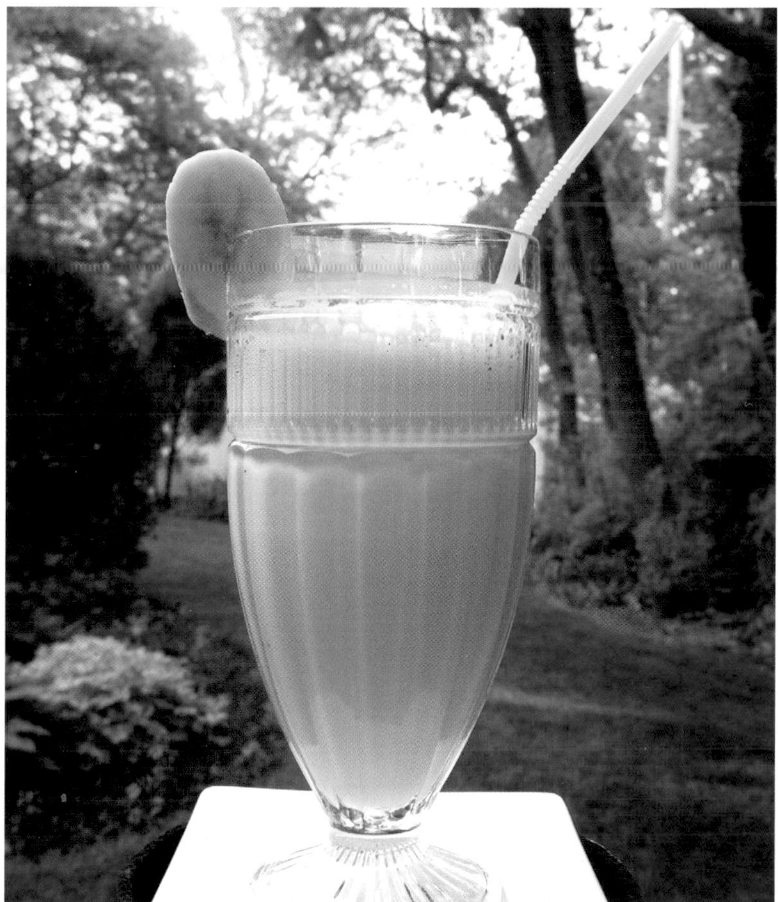

## Ingredients

½ cup ice
2 cups milk
2 bananas, ripe
1 cup yogurt
½ tsp fresh ginger, peeled and grated fine
2 Tbsp brown sugar or honey (optional)

## Directions

1. In a blender, add the ice, milk, yogurt, bananas, and ginger.
2. Blend until smooth.
3. Add sugar as needed.

**Notes** • *I use Lactaid (lactose-free) fat-free milk or 1% milk, but you can use any type of milk.* • *If you don't like ginger or there's none fresh, substitute ¼ tsp orange zest or vanilla or almond extract.* • *This smoothie is delicious and combines many of the best reflux foods.* • *Did you know that ginger in moderation is good for reflux? It packs a lot of flavor and is versatile as an ingredient in many dishes.*

# Gala Apple Honeydew Smoothie

*Serves 2*
***Nutritional information per serving***
Calories 114
Protein 2g
Carbohydrates 29g
Fat 0.5g

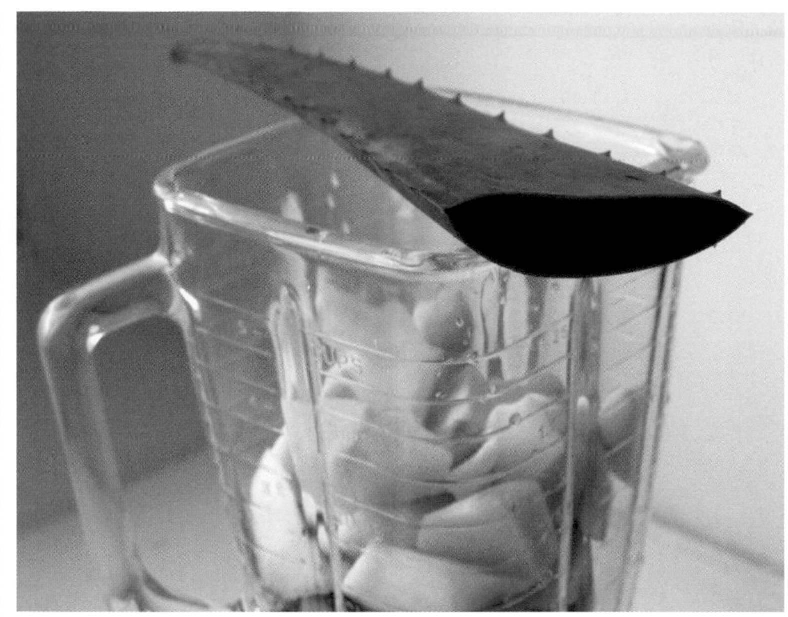

## Ingredients

2 cups honeydew melon (peeled, seeded, and cut into chunks)
4 Tbsp fresh aloe vera, skin removed
1 Gala apple (peeled, cored, and cut in half)
1/16 tsp lime zest (wash lime with warm water and use microplane to get the zest)
1½ cups ice
¼ tsp salt

## Directions

1. In a blender, add the melon, ice, aloe vera, apple, salt, and lime zest.
2. Begin blending on Pulse before switching to High. Stop and stir the mixture as needed to get a smooth consistency.

***Notes*** • *Aloe vera is good for reflux and gives this drink a nice, syrupy consistency. Don't eat the aloe plain—it doesn't have great flavor on its own.* • *Did you know that fruit becomes less acidic as it ripens? Store at room temperature for a week before using.* • *In addition to fresh aloe, you can buy it bottled—but fresh is better.* • *Aloe vera is readily available these days in markets and health-food stores, where they often sell it by the leaf so you don't have to buy the whole plant.* • *Every kitchen should have the handy little microplane for grating and zesting [see page 50].*

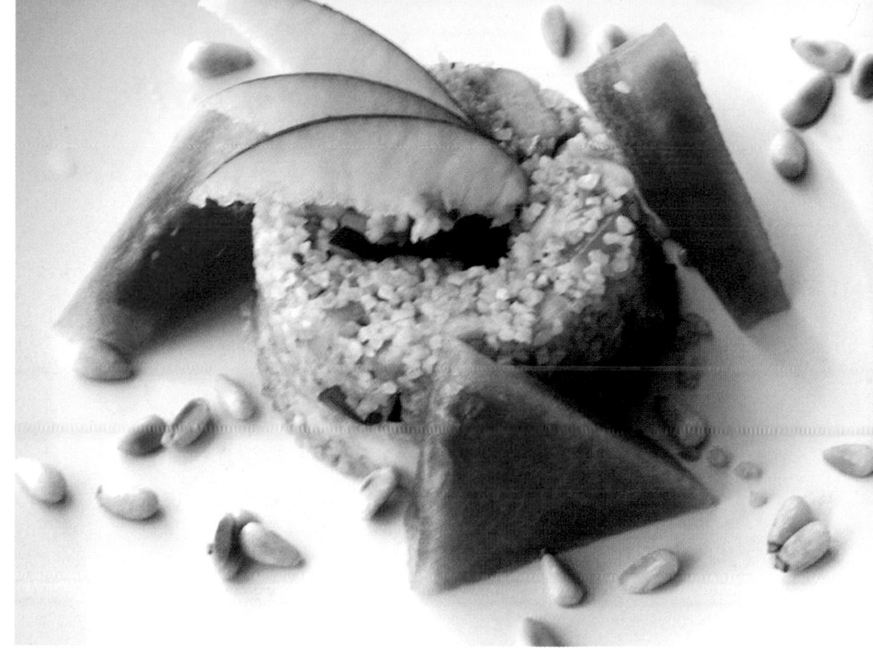

# Breakfast Couscous with Fruit and Pine Nuts

***Serves 3***
***Nutritional information per serving***
Calories 385
Protein 9g
Carbohydrates 86g
Fat 1g

### Ingredients

1 cup tabouli or other packaged couscous
1 banana (diced small)
1 apple (shredded with a grater)
1 cup orange juice
¼ tsp ginger (grated or microplaned)
2 Tbsp honey or raw sugar
2 Tbsp raisins
¼ tsp allspice
Salt to taste
1 tsp pine nuts, toasted

### Directions

1. Heat a pan over medium heat. Add the couscous and toast for a few minutes until it releases its aroma and turns golden brown. Place in a bowl.
2. Bring the orange juice to a simmer and pour over the couscous. Cover bowl tightly with plastic wrap and let sit for 5 minutes.
3. Stir the couscous with a fork to separate the grains.
4. When the couscous is cool or room temperature, add the banana, apple, ginger, raisins, allspice, salt, and honey or sugar. Stir to combine.
5. Place on a plate. Sprinkle with 1 tsp toasted pine nuts.

***Notes*** • *To serve this dish in the shape of a ring, spoon the final mixture into a small ring-mold. Pack the couscous tightly so it won't collapse when the mold is removed. Hold a serving plate upside down over the mold, invert them together quickly, and carefully remove the mold.* • *A few drops of orange juice can be added to the grated apples to prevent them from turning brown.* • *I prefer fresh orange juice when it is in season.* • *Orange juice by itself is too acidic for the reflux diet, but as an ingredient in this dish, the acidity is absorbed; the pH of this dish is 5.5.*

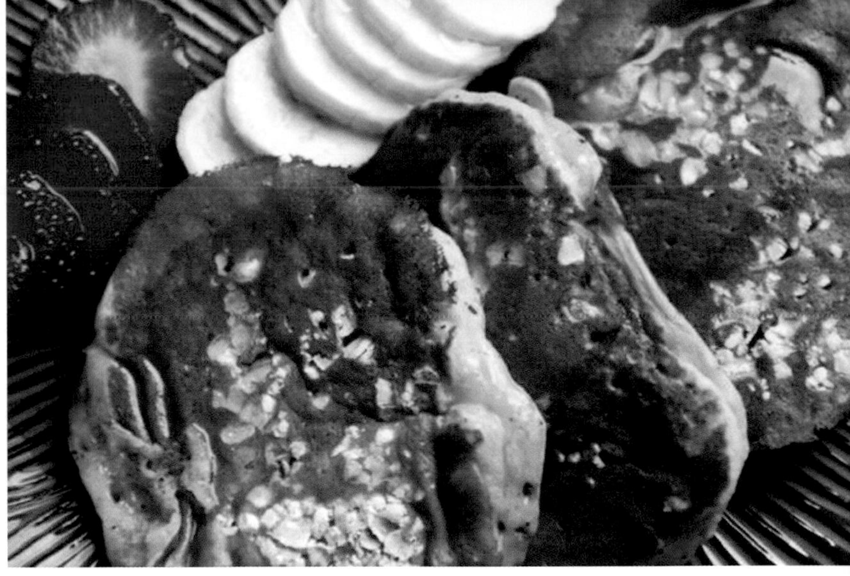

# OMG (Oh My God) Banana Oatmeal Pancakes

***Serves 4***
***Nutritional information per serving***
Calories 220
Protein 7g
Carbohydrates 36g
Fat 7g

## Ingredients

2 Tbsp light brown sugar
½ cup oat flour
½ cup all-purpose flour
1 tsp baking powder
½ tsp salt
⅛ tsp nutmeg
2 large eggs
3 bananas, blended or food processed
2 Tbsp (1 oz.) nonfat sour cream or buttermilk
Milk (to consistency)
1 Tbsp butter (for cooking)
Maple syrup, as desired

## Directions

1. Mix first six ingredients together in a bowl.
2. Whisk in the sour cream or buttermilk, the eggs, and the bananas.
3. If the mixture is too thick, add milk a few tablespoons at a time.
4. Preheat a nonstick pan over low to medium heat. Wipe a paper towel that has been rubbed with butter on the bottom of the pan. (Remove excess butter with the same paper towel and use again before cooking the next pancake.)
5. Using a ladle, pour some batter into the pan.
6. Flip pancake when the underside is golden brown, and cook until no longer wet inside.
7. Keep warm until all the pancakes are ready.
8. Serve with maple syrup, and can be topped with diced apples.

**Notes** • *I like to use Canadian D-grade maple syrup (equivalent of grade C in the U.S.) for its darker color and stronger flavor.* • *Cooking in a nonstick pan allows you to use butter sparingly.* • *You can make your own oat flour by blending rolled oats in a food processor or blender until fine.* • *If you make the batter the night before, don't add the baking powder until just before cooking. This batter will be slightly darker, but the result will be just as delicious.* • *Adding a tiny bit of diced mango to the batter just before cooking gives these pancakes a great flavor and pleasing color.*

# Crunchy-Wheat French Toast

*Serves 3 (2 slices per serving)*
***Nutritional information per serving***
Calories 212
Protein 9g
Carbohydrates 34g
Fat 4g

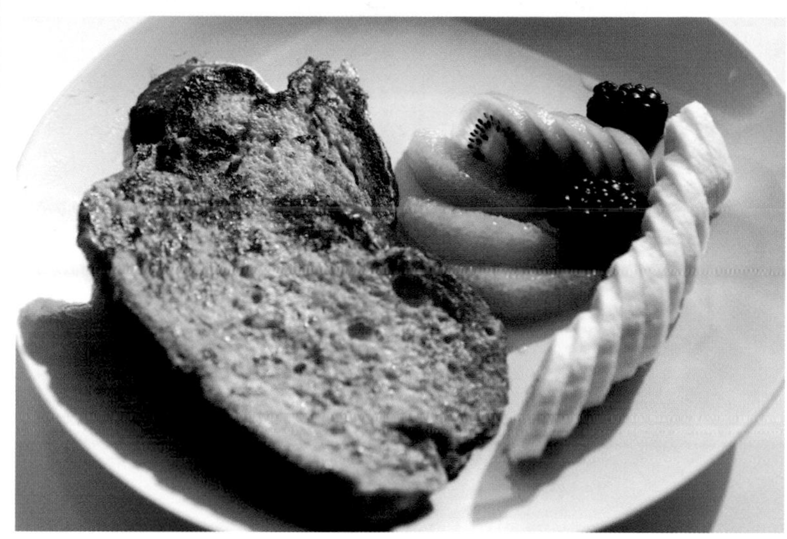

### Ingredients

6 slices white or challah bread
½ cup Total cereal (lightly crushed)
2 eggs
½ cup milk
½ cup flavored yogurt (I like raspberry)
¼ tsp vanilla extract
2 Tbsp brown sugar
1 Tbsp butter (or pan spray)
Salt to taste
Honey or maple syrup, to taste

### Directions

1. In a bowl, whisk the eggs, vanilla extract, brown sugar, yogurt, and milk.
2. Place two slices of bread in the bowl, without overlapping.
3. As the slices become saturated with the custard, flip them over.
4. Preheat a nonstick pan over medium heat. Wipe a paper towel that has been rubbed with butter on the bottom of the pan.
5. Sprinkle pan with a third of the cereal, and add the bread.
6. Cook until both sides are golden brown. Repeat directions for the remaining slices of bread.
7. Serve with syrup or honey.

**Notes** • *If you use English muffins, you don't need to put salt in the custard. • I like using challah bread for this dish—it reminds me of brioche without all the fat, and it tastes like cake. You can use any bread, but slice it if it's dense. For example, I slice bagels into thirds or thinner.*

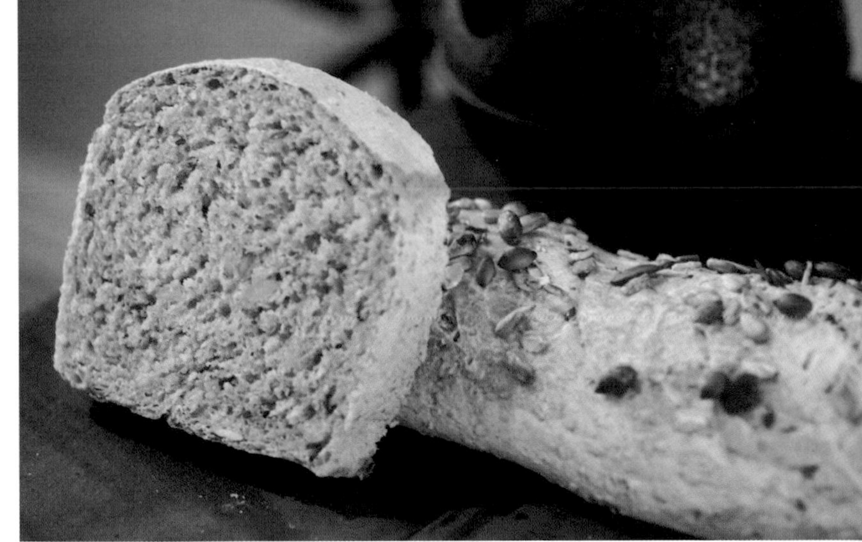

# Marc's Homemade 5-Grain Bread

***Makes 20 slices***
***Nutritional information per serving***
Calories 91
Protein 3g
Carbohydrates 17g
Fat 2g

### Ingredients

3 cups all-purpose flour
1 cup whole-wheat flour
1¼ cups water
1 tsp dry yeast or ½ oz fresh yeast
2 tsp honey
2 Tbsp sesame seeds
2 Tbsp pumpkin seeds
2 Tbsp flaxseeds
2 Tbsp sunflower seeds
2 Tbsp rolled oats
2 tsp salt

### Directions

1. Soak the sesame, pumpkin, flax, rolled oats, and sunflower seeds in warm water for 20 minutes. Drain.
2. Mix the two flours with the water, yeast, and honey for 2 minutes in a mixer (using the bread attachment hook). Let sit for 20 minutes.
3. Add the salt and soaked seeds. Mix for another 5 minutes. Cover and let rest for 15 minutes at a minimum temperature of 72°F.
4. Turn out onto a floured work surface.
5. Shape into an 8-inch loaf by first flattening the dough into a rectangle about 8x5 inches, then rolling it up toward the 8-inch side.
6. Place in an 8-inch loaf pan that has been oiled or sprayed with nonstick spray.
7. Cover with parchment paper or an oiled sheet of aluminum foil and keep warm, about 72–77°F, until the dough doubles in volume and comes to the top of the pan.
8. Remove the parchment paper or aluminum foil.
9. Place in a convection oven at 400°F, or in a conventional oven at 425°F, and cook for 20–25 minutes or until the crust is golden brown.
10. Remove from pan immediately.
11. Let sit for 15 minutes and enjoy for a healthy breakfast or with a meal.

***Notes*** • *The dough should rest 20 minutes to rehydrate the flour.* • *This bread can be kept fresh for two or three days in a paper bag, or frozen in individual slices to make a toaster snack.* • *If you prefer a darker color to the bread, increase the oven temperature about 25 degrees.* • *You can make two loaves at once and freeze the second.* • *Don't forget to let the bread cool before eating. After cooking, the water continues to evaporate; when cooled, the bread will be lighter in texture.*

# Healthy Raisin Bran Muffins

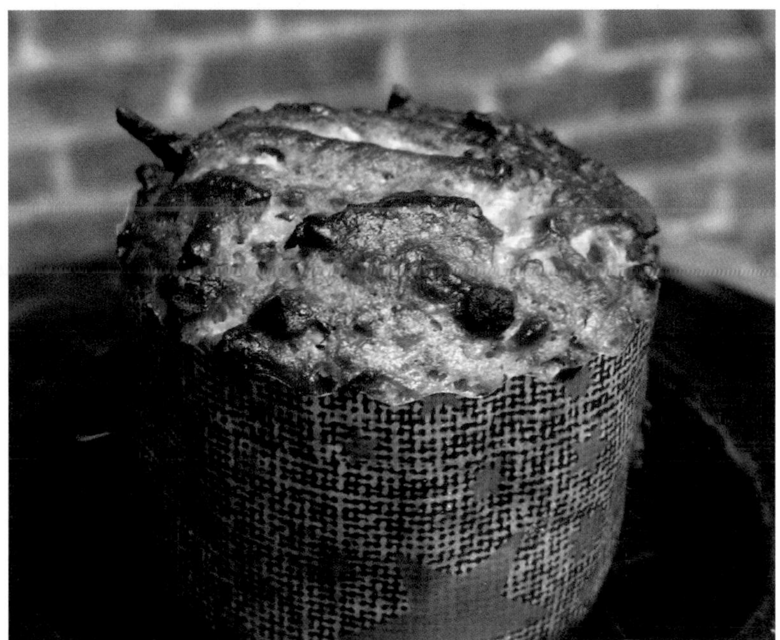

***Serves 4 (1 muffin per serving)***
***Nutritional information per serving***
Calories 171
Protein 5g
Carbohydrates 35g
Fat 3g

## Ingredients

- 2 Tbsp dark raisins or dried noncitrus fruit of your choice
- ¼ cup whole milk (you can use lower-fat milk if you desire)
- 1 egg
- ⅓ cup yogurt
- 1 Tbsp milled flaxseed
- 3 Tbsp brown sugar
- ⅓ cup bran cereal
- ½ cup all purpose flour
- 1½ tsp baking powder
- Salt to taste
- ½ Golden Delicious or Gala apple (washed and grated, including the skin)

## Directions

1. Using a small saucepan, bring the milk to a boil and pour over the raisins.
2. In a bowl, mix the flaxseed, sugar, cereal, flour, baking powder, and salt.
3. In a separate bowl, whisk the egg, apple, milk mixture, and yogurt.
4. Add the egg mixture to the dry ingredients with a whisk.
5. Pour mixture into muffin molds that have been buttered or sprayed with a nonstick spray or lined with paper cups.
6. Cook at 350°F for 15 to 20 minutes or until golden brown.
7. Let cool a few minutes.

**Notes** • *Extra muffins can be frozen in a plastic bag.* • *To reheat, cut in half and heat in the oven until golden brown, or use them to make French toast.* • *If you are unable to find milled flaxseed, purchase whole flaxseed and grind in a spice mill or coffee grinder.* • *It's easy to recognize when the muffins are ready. The top of the muffin expands and the fissures turn golden brown as the mixture caramelizes.* • *Raisins by themselves are acidic, but they can be used in dishes like this one, or in cereal with milk or with oatmeal, because there is buffering of the acid.*

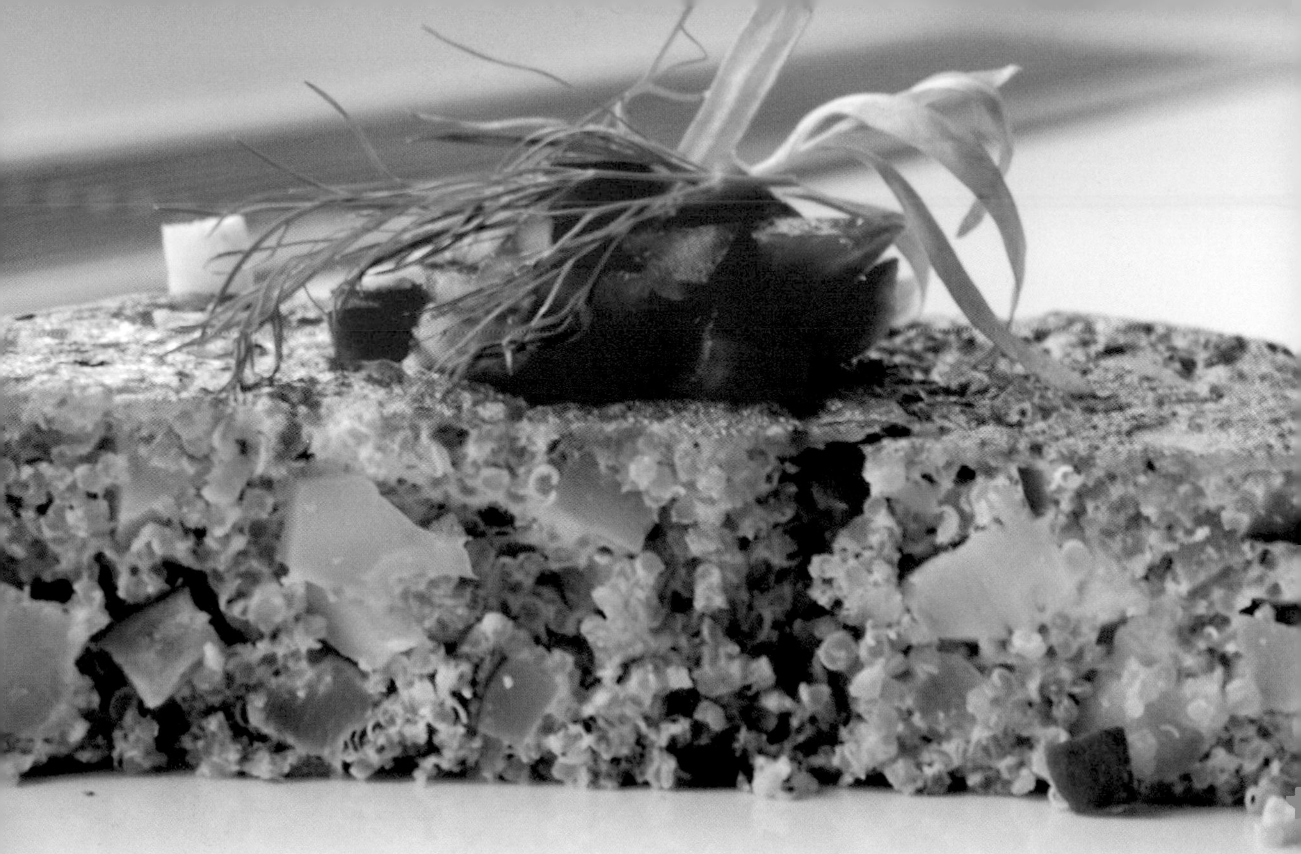

*Serves 6*
***Nutritional information per serving***
Calories 138
Protein 8g
Carbohydrates 18g
Fat 5g

# Vegetable Frittata with Quinoa

## Directions

1. Heat the oven to 375°F.
2. Pour the chicken stock in a saucepan and add the parsnips. When parsnips are thoroughly cooked, remove them and reserve the stock.
3. Add the cauliflower to the stock and cook thoroughly. Remove cauliflower and reserve the stock.
4. Add the zucchini to the stock and cook thoroughly before removing.
5. Heat the stock again and add the quinoa. Bring to a boil and cook about 5 minutes or until al dente. Remove the quinoa from the stock.
6. Place all of the cooked vegetables, quinoa, diced tomato, herbs, and Roquefort in a large bowl. Mix until the cheese combines completely with the other ingredients.
7. In a small bowl, whisk the eggs with a fork until whites and yolks are mixed.

### Ingredients

1 cup parsnips (peeled and diced into roughly ½-inch cubes)
1 cup cauliflower, broken into florets
1 cup zucchini, cut into roughly ½-inch slices
½ cup red plum tomato (cored and diced)
½ cup quinoa
4 eggs
2 tsp Herbes de Provence
2 tsp Roquefort (or other blue cheese)
2 cups chicken stock (no MSG, low sodium)

8. Add the eggs to the vegetable mixture and stir gently.
9. Rub 1 tsp of butter on the bottom of a 10-inch nonstick ovenproof pan (or coat with a nonstick spray).
10. Heat the pan on the stovetop. When the butter is frothy, lower the temperature to medium-low and add the frittata mixture. Cook for a few minutes and finish in the oven until done to your taste. (I like them slightly runny for the velvety texture.)
11. Flip onto a plate by holding the plate upside down on top of the pan and flipping pan and plate together.
12. You can brush the top of the frittata with melted butter and serve with toast.

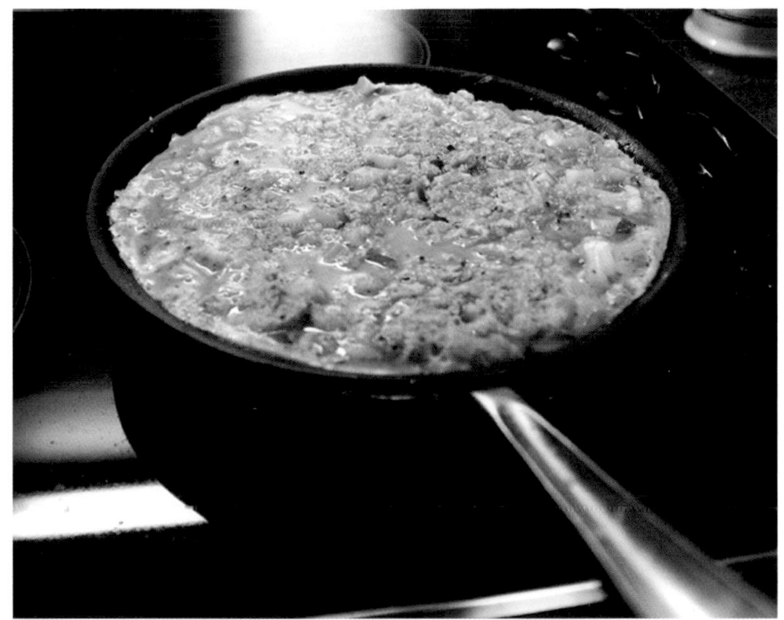

***Notes*** • *If you can't find any Herbes de Provence, mix equal parts thyme, oregano, marjoram, basil, and sage.* • *Cooking zucchini in the stock until softened should take about one minute. Parsnips and cauliflower take five to seven minutes to reach a perfect "al dente."* • *The chicken stock or broth can be kept and reused, since it has been enriched with flavor and vitamins from the vegetables* • *The grain quinoa (pronounced KEEN-wah) is a complete protein that contains all the essential amino acids, but without the cholesterol found in animal proteins.*

# Omelet with Fine Herbs and Whole-Wheat Toast

*Serves 2*
*Nutritional information per serving*
Calories 234
Protein 14g
Carbohydrates 14g
Fat 14g

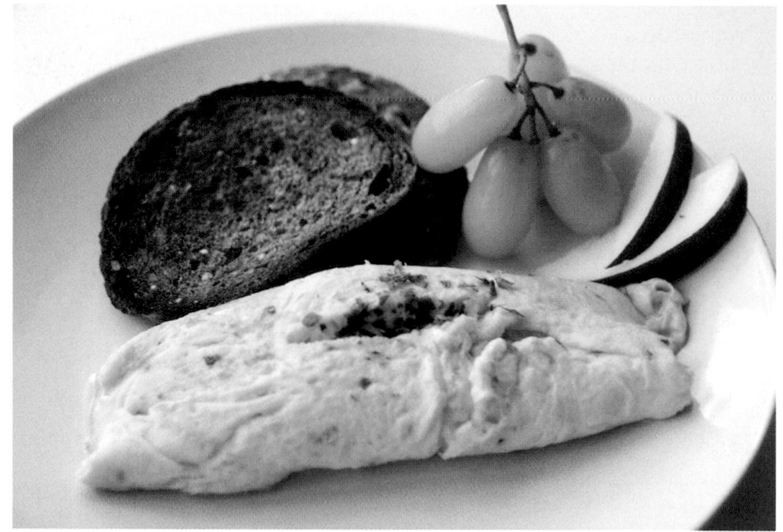

## Ingredients

4 eggs
4 sprigs parsley (washed, dried, stems removed, chopped fine)
1 sprig tarragon (washed, dried, stems removed, chopped fine)
1 sprig thyme (washed, dried, stems removed, chopped fine)
2 tsp water or nonfat sour cream
2 tsp butter
Salt to taste

## Directions

1. Whisk 2 of the eggs with a fork. (You will make two small omelets, two eggs each.)
2. Add the water or nonfat sour cream, along with the herbs and salt.
3. Preheat an 8-inch nonstick pan on medium heat.
4. Add the butter and cook until it froths and turns slightly brown.
5. Immediately add the egg mixture.
6. Let the eggs coagulate for a few seconds, then remove from heat while stirring with a wooden spoon or high-heat rubber spatula.
7. Return to the heat and bang the pan gently to remove air bubbles. Lower the temperature.
8. Using a nonstick spatula, fold one third of the omelet to the middle.
9. Fold the other third, slightly overlapping the middle, and flip carefully onto a plate. Repeat steps for next omelet.
10. You can brush the top with a little melted butter (optional).
11. Sprinkle with a few more herbs and serve toast on the side.

*Serves 2*
***Nutritional information per serving***
Calories 188
Protein 14g
Carbohydrates 2g
Fat 14g

# Delish Mushroom Omelet

### Ingredients

4 eggs
3 domestic mushrooms, about the size of a silver dollar (washed, dried, cut in half to form two half spheres, then placed flat-side down and sliced thin)
4 sprigs parsley (washed, dried, stems removed, chopped fine)
2 tsp water or nonfat sour cream
2 tsp butter
Salt to taste

### Directions

1. Whisk the eggs with a fork.
2. Add the water or nonfat sour cream, parsley, and salt.
3. Preheat an 8-inch nonstick pan on medium heat.
4. Spray the pan with nonstick spray. Add the mushrooms to the pan and spread evenly. When they are golden brown on one side, season with salt, flip, and cook the other side until tender. Reserve the mushrooms on paper to absorb excess moisture and oil.
5. Wipe the pan clean with a paper towel and preheat on medium heat.
6. Add most of the butter (save a bit if you need for second omelet) and cook until it froths and turns slightly brown.
7. Immediately add half the egg mixture. (Repeat directions for the second omelet.)
8. Let the eggs coagulate for a few seconds. Remove from heat while stirring with a wooden spoon or high-heat rubber spatula.
9. Return to the heat and bang the pan gently on the stove to remove air bubbles. Lower the temperature.
10. When the mixture is almost set (it should not have any color), slide the omelet to the edge of the pan. Place almost half the reserved mushrooms in the center of the omelet.
11. Fold one third of the omelet to the middle with a nonstick spatula.
12. Fold the other third slightly overlapping the middle, and carefully flip onto a plate.
13. You can brush the top with a little melted butter (optional).
14. Sprinkle with some of the mushrooms and serve toast on the side. Repeat for second omelet.

**Notes** • *You can use any variety of mushrooms. I love the flavor of shitake mushrooms, but remember to remove their tough stems.* • *Mushrooms cook best in a large pan and spread in a single layer. If the mushrooms are overcrowded, the water they yield will make them boil instead of sauté.*

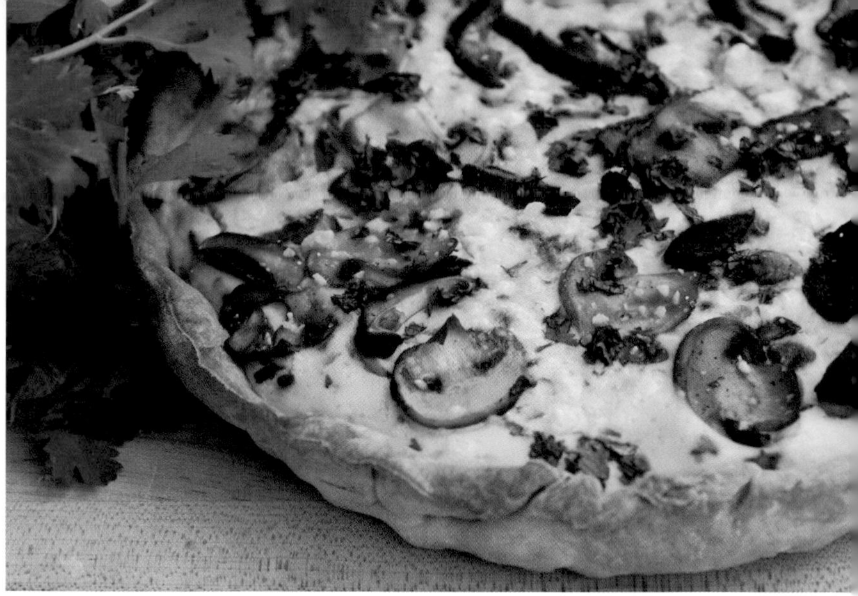

# Quench-the-Fire Quiche with Tofu and Mushrooms

***Serves 6***
***Nutritional information per serving***
Calories 292
Protein 12g
Carbohydrates 77g
Fat 10g

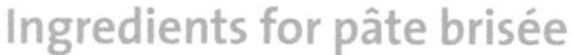

### Ingredients for pâte brisée

- 1¾ cups all-purpose flour
- 5 Tbsp water
- 2 Tbsp butter
- 1 egg yolk
- Salt to taste

### Ingredients for custard

- 1 cup (6 oz) silken tofu, soft
- ½ cup of the water from the tofu
- 2 egg yolks
- Salt to taste
- 2 Tbsp Parmesan cheese

### Ingredients for assembling

- 1½ cups (4 oz) shitake mushrooms (stems removed, washed, and cut into thin strips)
- ½ cup dry porcini mushrooms (rehydrated in cold water for an hour, drained)
- 1½ cups (4 oz) domestic mushrooms (remove ¼ inch from the stem and slice thin)
- 1 Tbsp butter
- ¼ tsp grated nutmeg
- 2 Tbsp chopped parsley or cilantro

### Directions for the custard

1. Place the tofu and water in a blender and process until smooth.
2. Add the 2 egg yolks and the Parmesan cheese.
3. Season with salt to taste.

### Directions for the pâte brisée and assembling

1. In a glass or plastic measuring cup, combine the water, butter, and salt.
2. Melt the butter and let it cool.
3. In a bowl, add the flour, 1 egg yolk, and the mixture of water, salt, and butter.
4. Use a plastic scraper to cut the butter into the flour.
5. When the mixture is completely combined, form into a circle about 1 inch thick and 6 inches in diameter.
6. Wrap in plastic wrap and refrigerate for 30 minutes.
7. Spray the inside of an 8-inch tart mold with nonstick spray, or rub with butter. Roll out the dough on a well-floured flat surface until the diameter is about 2 inches larger than the tart mold all the way around and the same thickness throughout.
8. Place the dough in the mold and refrigerate for 20 minutes or until dough is leathery.

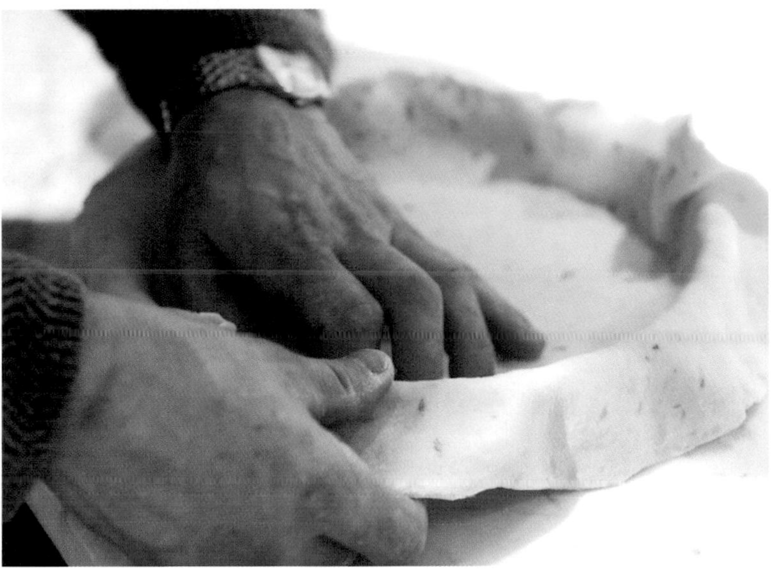

9. Place parchment paper or aluminum foil on the cold tart shell and fill tart with dried beans or special metal balls used for "blind baking" (prebaking).
10. Cook in the oven at 350°F for 10–15 minutes or until the dough becomes chalky.
11. Remove the beans or special balls as well as the parchment paper or aluminum foil.
12. Return to the oven until the dough is golden brown.
13. Allow to cool.
14. Sauté the mushrooms in butter and a little bit of salt until all the moisture from them is released and they turn golden brown.
15. Add the sautéed mushrooms to the bottom of the cooked tart.
16. Cover with the tofu custard.
17. Sprinkle with chopped parsley or cilantro and nutmeg.
18. Return to the oven until custard sets and top is golden brown, approximately 30 minutes.
19. Serve immediately.

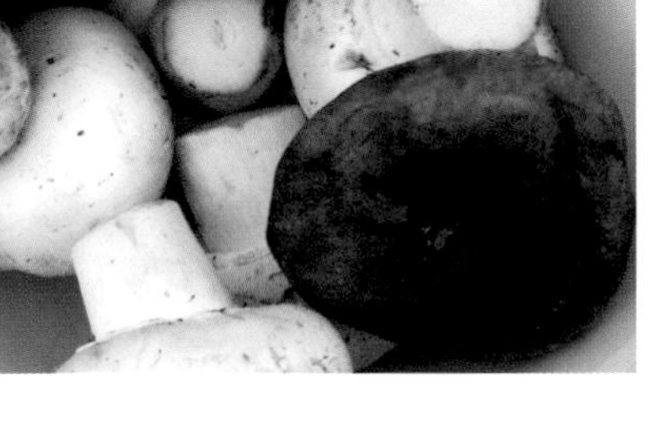

***Notes*** • *Place the finished quiche under the broiler for a short time to get a nice golden color on top.* • *The dough can be prepared a day or two ahead and covered with plastic wrap or sealed in a plastic bag.* • *Instead of mixing the dough by hand, it can be made in a food processor by pulsing all the ingredients together 10–15 seconds.*

## By-the-Rules Oatmeal

*Serves 2*
*Nutritional information per serving*
Calories 185
Protein 8g
Carbohydrates 32g
Fat 4g

### Ingredients

1 cup oatmeal (3 oz steel cut oats, also called Irish oats)
½ cup whole milk
1½ cups boiling water
½ tsp salt

### Directions

1. Mix the oatmeal in a saucepan with the milk to form a paste.
2. Add the boiling water and salt. Mix with a wooden spoon and bring to a boil. Stir often to avoid burning the bottom.
3. Simmer 10–15 minutes, stirring occasionally.

**Notes** • *Don't worry too much about the fat content of the whole milk. There's less than 4 grams of fat in 4 fl oz.* • *To shorten the cooking time, use rolled or instant oats.* • *For a nutty flavor, toast the oats first. To add this step, toast them in a pan on the stovetop or in the oven until they turn slightly darker and have a nutty smell.*

## Oatmeal Marc's Way

*Serves 2*
*Nutritional information per serving*
Calories 323
Protein 10g
Carbohydrates 61g
Fat 1g

### Ingredients

1 cup oatmeal (3 oz, rolled or instant, toasted)
1 cup milk
⅓ tsp salt
½ tsp vanilla extract
Pinch of nutmeg (remember, it's strong!)
4 Tbsp light brown sugar, packed

### Directions

1. Bring the milk to a boil in a saucepan.
2. Add the salt, oatmeal, vanilla extract, nutmeg, and sugar.
3. Return to a simmer while stirring.
4. Cook 5 minutes. (Cooking time depends on type and brand of oatmeal.)

**Notes** • *Use dark brown sugar if you like a stronger molasses taste.* • *The brown sugar can be replaced with honey or maple syrup.* • *If you don't often use oats, keep them in a sealed container either in the refrigerator or a cool dry place.* • *Did you know that using instant or rolled oats shortens the cooking time? They have already been steamed, cut small, and rolled.*

*Serves 2*
***Nutritional information per serving***
Calories 490
Protein 11g
Carbohydrates 107g
Fat 1g

# Muesli-Style Oatmeal

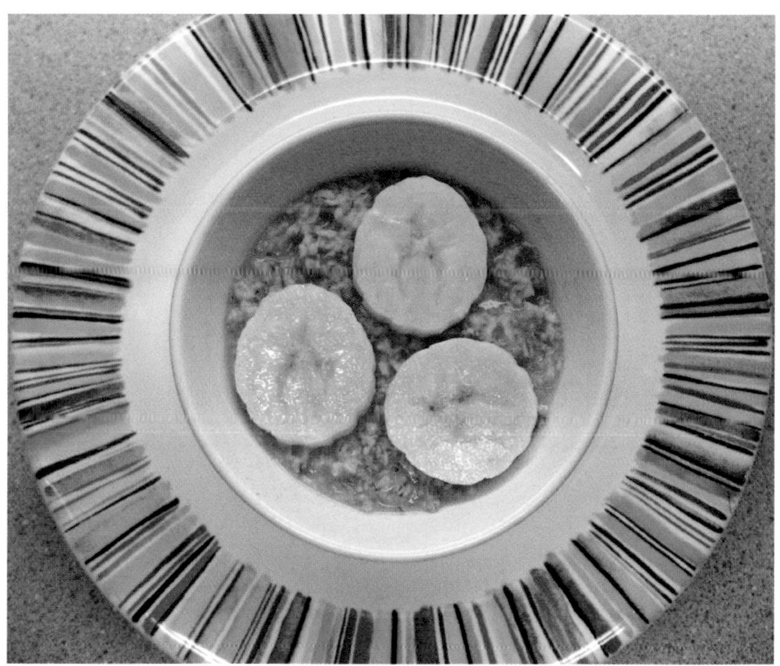

### Ingredients

- 1 cup instant oatmeal
- 1 cup milk
- 2 Tbsp raisins (covered with water, brought to a boil and drained)
- ½ banana, diced or sliced
- ½ golden apple, peeled and diced
- Pinch of salt
- 2 tsp sugar or honey

### Directions

1. The evening before (or at least two hours before), mix the oatmeal, milk, raisins, salt, and sugar (or honey) together in a bowl.
2. Cover and place in the refrigerator.
3. Add the fruit just before serving.
4. If the mix is too thick, add milk as needed.

***Notes*** • *I first came across muesli at Curtain Bluff Resort in Antigua, courtesy of Chef Christophe Blatz. (He is Alsatian, from the Alsace region of France bordering Germany and Switzerland.) His delicious muesli inspired this recipe, although I have removed the heavy cream.* • *This oatmeal is not cooked, but is left overnight in the refrigerator to rehydrate.* • *Dark raisins or golden raisins (or a mix of both) can be used.* • *Use any combination of fruit (except citrus or blueberries).* • *This makes a delicious breakfast during the summer, although it's delicious any time of year!* • *The apple can be grated instead of diced.*

# Instant Polenta with Sesame Seeds

*Serves 3*
***Nutritional information per serving***
Calories 280
Protein 9g
Carbohydrates 49g
Fat 6g

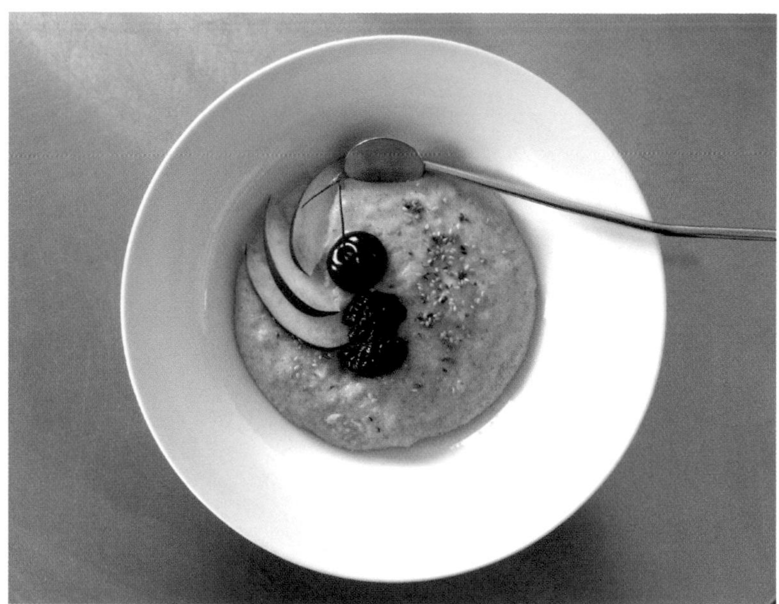

### Ingredients

- ¾ cup instant polenta or corn meal
- 3 cups whole milk (or lower-fat milk if you prefer)
- 3 Tbsp brown sugar
- 1 tsp orange extract
- ½ tsp vanilla extract
- Salt to taste
- 1 Tbsp sesame seeds (toast slowly in a pan until golden brown)

### Directions

1. Bring the milk to a boil.
2. Add the polenta or corn meal and whisk vigorously to prevent lumps.
3. Cook until you get a creamy consistency.
4. Add the sugar, salt, and vanilla and orange extract just before serving.
5. Serve in a bowl and sprinkle with sesame seeds.

***Notes*** • *When you buy corn meal or polenta, look for instant or 5-minute versions to save cooking time.* • *Orange extract can be replaced by adding a strip of orange peel (washed and removed with a peeler) to the simmering milk for a couple of minutes. Remove the peel and proceed to Step 2.* • *This dish uses sesame seeds, which are filled with oil. Their flavor contrasts superbly with the note of orange.*

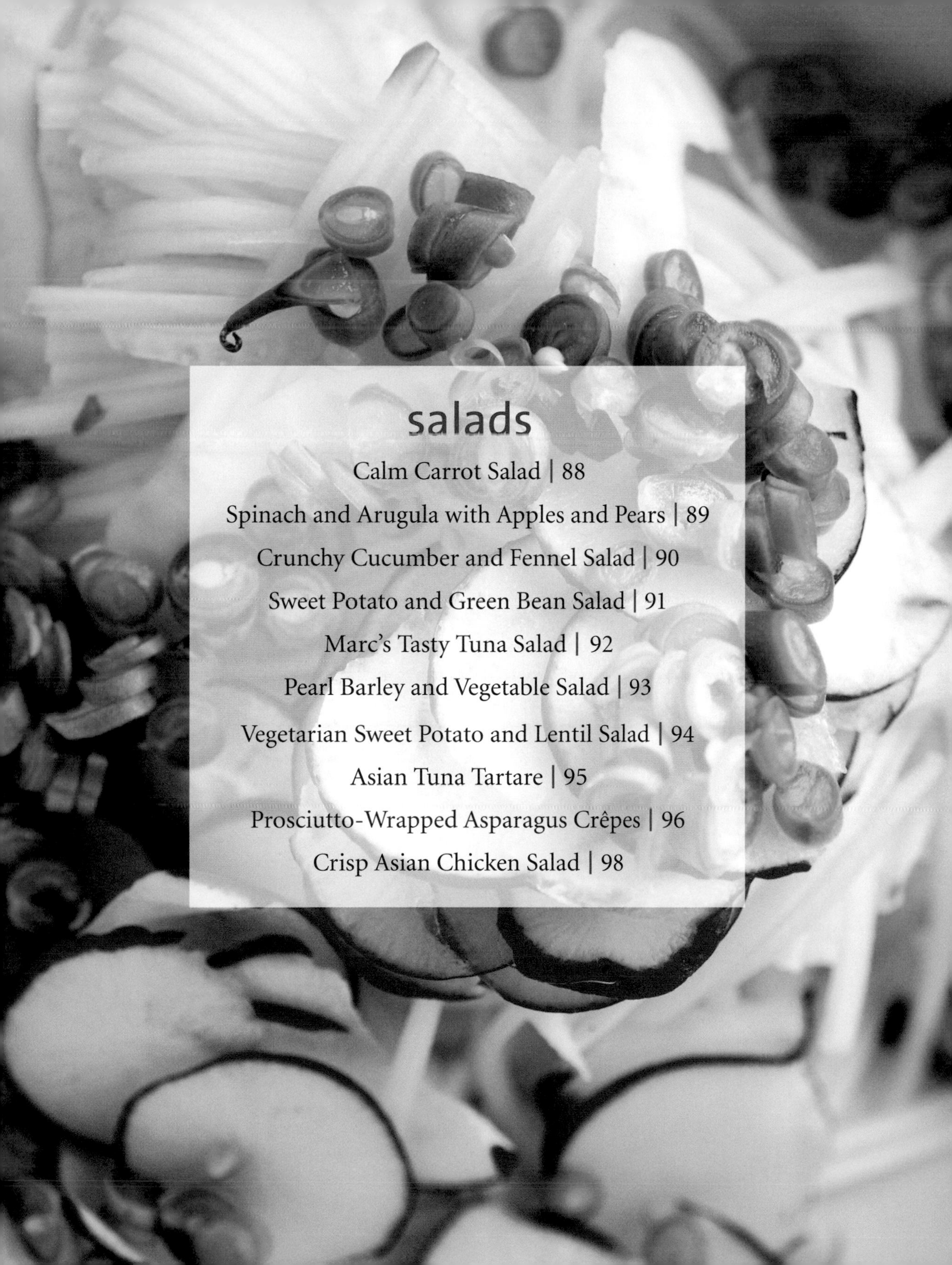

# salads


Calm Carrot Salad | 88

Spinach and Arugula with Apples and Pears | 89

Crunchy Cucumber and Fennel Salad | 90

Sweet Potato and Green Bean Salad | 91

Marc's Tasty Tuna Salad | 92

Pearl Barley and Vegetable Salad | 93

Vegetarian Sweet Potato and Lentil Salad | 94

Asian Tuna Tartare | 95

Prosciutto-Wrapped Asparagus Crêpes | 96

Crisp Asian Chicken Salad | 98

# Calm Carrot Salad

*Serves 2*
*Nutritional information per serving*
Calories 236
Protein 3g
Carbohydrates 46g
Fat 5g

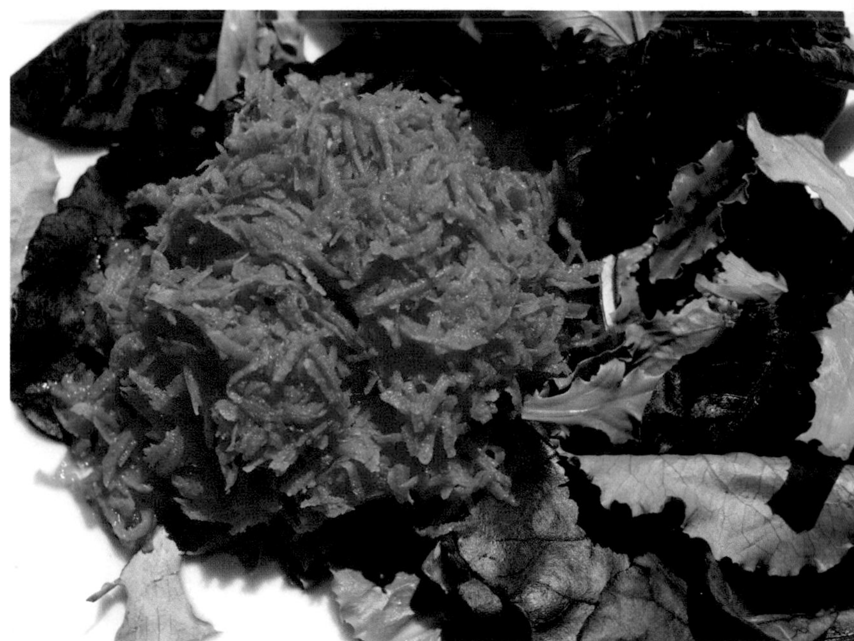

## Ingredients

1 lb carrots (peeled, trimmed, and grated)
¼ lb mesclun greens
2 Tbsp raisins
2 Tbsp orange juice
1 tsp dried oregano
2 Tbsp brown sugar
2 tsp olive oil
¼ tsp salt

## Directions

1. In a bowl, mix the raisins, orange juice, oregano, brown sugar, olive oil, and salt. Let sit for about 5 minutes.
2. Pour the dressing over the carrots and mix thoroughly.
3. Season with additional salt, as needed.
4. Serve over a few mesclun leaves.

***Notes*** • *The infusion of oregano into the orange juice brings out its flavor.*

***Serves 3***
***Nutritional information per serving***
Calories 83
Protein 2g
Carbohydrates 18g
Fat 1g

# Spinach and Arugula with Apples and Pears

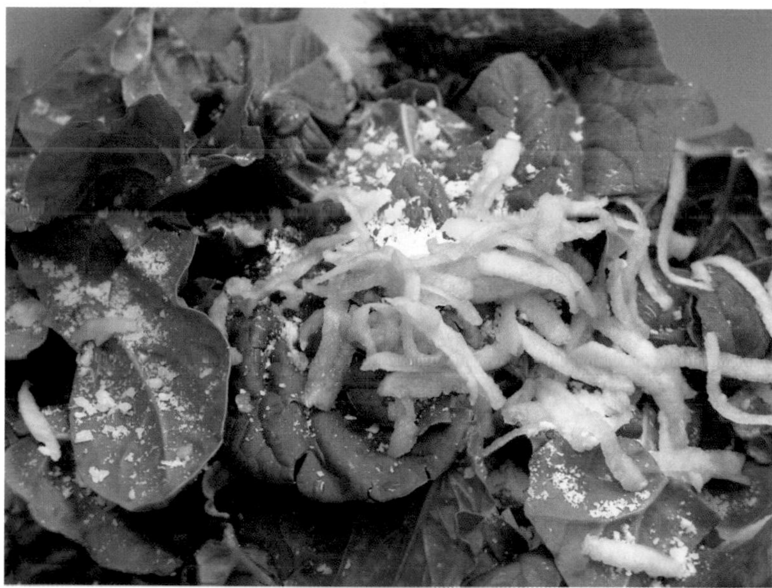

### Ingredients

2 cups spinach
1 cup arugula
3 Tbsp orange juice
1 Golden Delicious or red apple (peeled and grated on a coarse grater)
1 pear (peeled and diced to ½-inch cubes)
1 Tbsp Parmesan cheese, grated
1 tsp sesame seeds, toasted
Salt to taste

### Directions

1. Pour the orange juice over the apples and pears to keep them from turning brown (it slows the oxidation process).
2. Wash the spinach and arugula several times until clean. One way is to use a salad spinner. Another is to plunge the greens into a large bowl filled with cold water, remove, and repeat as needed. Keep washing until you no longer see sand on the bottom of the bowl.
3. Dry thoroughly; a salad spinner is easiest.
4. Toast the sesame seeds in a pan on the stovetop or in the oven until golden brown. Transfer them to a bowl or plate immediately to avoid burning.
5. Mix the spinach, arugula, apple, pear, Parmesan cheese, orange juice, and salt.
6. Present on a plate and sprinkle with sesame seeds.

***Notes*** • *This salad can be served with sesame sticks or toasted whole-wheat bread.*

# Crunchy Cucumber and Fennel Salad

*Serves 2*
***Nutritional information per serving***
Calories 88
Protein 5g
Carbohydrates 18g
Fat 1g

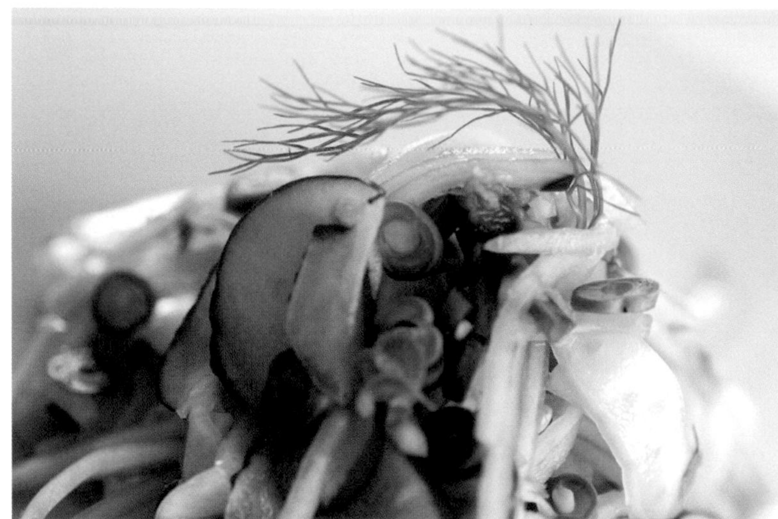

## Ingredients

- 1 cup cucumber (peeled and seeded)
- 1 cup fennel (peel off any brown or dehydrated sides, slice thin)
- 5 green beans (cut into thin slices)
- 4 radishes (cut into thin slices)
- 2 Tbsp fish sauce (Thai nam pla sauce)
- 1 Tbsp ginger
- 4 Tbsp apple juice
- 2 Tbsp oyster sauce
- 10 leaves tarragon (chopped coarse)

## Directions

1. Cut a small piece of cucumber; wrap the rest and keep refrigerated.
2. Peel and shred with a coarse grater.
3. Slice the fennel thin with a mandoline slicer or a box grater (on the side allowing slicing).

## For the dressing

1. In a bowl, add the fish sauce, ginger, apple juice, oyster sauce, and tarragon.
2. Use immediately or keep up to two hours.

## For presentation

1. In a bowl, place the fennel, cucumber, radishes, and half of the green beans.
2. Pour the dressing on top and mix, using a pair of tongs.
3. Serve on a platter or individual plates.
4. Sprinkle with the rest of the cut green beans.

**Notes** • *Using a mandoline, box grater, or food processor results in even cuts and gives the salad a pleasing texture. If a mandoline or box grater is not available, cut the fennel bulb in half lengthwise, place the flat side down on a cutting board, and cut into thin slices.* • *A food processor with a slicing disc could also be used.* • *I love this salad in the summer, even though fennel and cucumber are available all year round. It is a nice, light salad with no fat and plenty of flavor. The green beans and radish give it splashes of color.*

# Sweet Potato and Green Bean Salad

***Serves 6***
***Nutritional information per serving***
Calories 253
Protein 3g
Carbohydrates 39g
Fat 10g

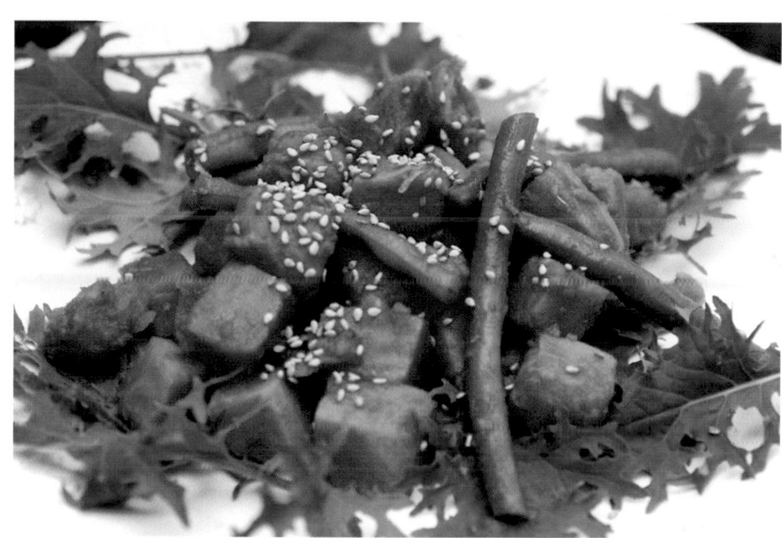

## Ingredients

1 lb green beans (both ends removed, cut into pieces about 2 inches long)
1 lb sweet potatoes (peeled and cut into 1-inch cubes)
2 Tbsp olive oil
Zest from 1 lemon (washed, to yield about 2 tsp)
¼ cup maple syrup
1 cup pineapple juice
½ tsp ground cumin
2 bay leaves
2 Tbsp soy sauce
1 tsp sesame seeds
3 cups baby arugula or watercress

## Directions

1. Place the green beans in boiling salted water and cook until al dente. Remove and place in ice-cold water. Drain.
2. Place the pineapple juice, cumin, and bay leaves in a small saucepan. Simmer on low heat and reduce by half.
3. In a bowl, mix the maple syrup, pineapple juice reduction, and soy sauce.
4. Place the olive oil in a pan over high heat, add the sweet potatoes, and cook until golden brown on all sides.
5. Place the sweet potatoes in a bowl and add the green beans, lemon zest, maple and pineapple dressing. Toss until mixed.
6. Place the arugula (or watercress) on the bottom of a plate and the vegetables on top. Sprinkle with the toasted sesame seeds.
7. Serve immediately.

***Notes*** • *It is important to chill the green beans in ice-cold water immediately after cooking, or they will lose their bright green color.* • *Mixing the dressing with the sweet potatoes while they are still warm allows even distribution of the dressing throughout the salad.* • *The salad should be served at room temperature. If the potatoes are too warm, the watercress will wilt.*

# Marc's Tasty Tuna Salad

***Serves 4***
***Nutritional information per serving***
Calories 303
Protein 24g
Carbohydrates 33g
Fat 8g

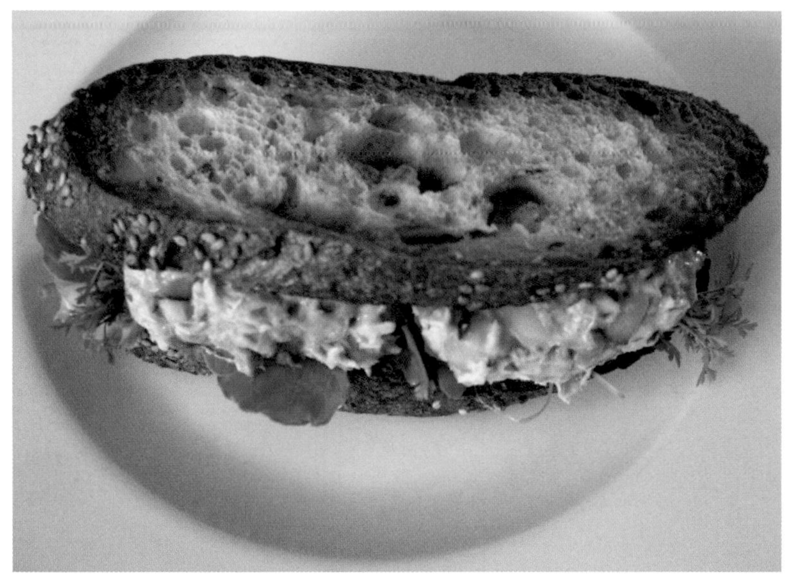

## Ingredients

- 10 oz canned tuna in water, drained
- ½ celery stalk (cut into ½-inch pieces)
- ½ cup cucumber (washed, cut in half lengthwise, seeds removed, cut into ¼-inch-wide strips and cut into ¼-inch pieces)
- ¼ cup carrots (peeled and shredded or chopped fine)
- 2½ Tbsp mayonnaise
- 2 Tbsp parsley (leaves removed, washed, dried, chopped fine, and washed again)
- 1 Tbsp capers (chopped fine)
- 3 anchovy filets (soaked in water for 5 minutes to remove excess salt, and drained)
- Lettuce leaves (arugula or watercress, washed and dried)
- ¼ tsp salt (or more), to taste
- 8 slices of bread, toasted

## Directions

1. In a bowl, mix the tuna, celery, cucumber, carrots, mayonnaise, salt, parsley, capers, and anchovies.
2. Place a few leaves of your favorite lettuce on the toast, add a portion of the salad, cover each sandwich with another slice of toast, and serve.

***Notes*** • *The anchovies and capers underscore the delicious flavor of the tuna.* • *Hellmann's mayonnaise is a good option, as it only has 1 gram of fat per tablespoon.* • *The chopped parsley should be washed twice, once before cutting and once after. The first washing removes any grit, and the second washing removes the excess chlorophyll, which otherwise stains the tuna salad green.*

# Pearl Barley and Vegetable Salad

***Serves 8***
***Nutritional information per serving***
Calories 129
Protein 4g
Carbohydrates 21g
Fat 4g

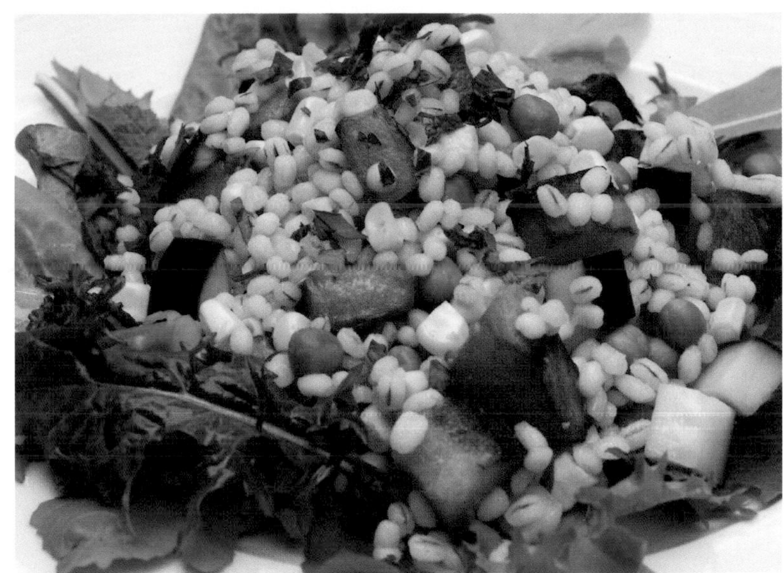

## Ingredients

- 3 cups baby greens loosely packed or ½ head Boston lettuce (washed and dried)
- 1 cup barley
- 2 cups chicken stock
- 1 cup corn (kernels removed from the cob)
- 2 cups butternut squash (skin removed and cut into ½-inch pieces)
- 1 cup peas
- 1 cup broccoli (cut into florets)
- 1 cup cucumber (washed, cut in half, seeds removed, and cut into ½-inch pieces)
- ½ cup chopped parsley (stems removed, washed, dried, and chopped fine)
- 2 Tbsp olive oil
- 1 tsp ginger, grated fine
- ½ cup green tea
- ½ cup peach juice

## Directions

1. In a medium saucepan over medium heat, cook the barley in the chicken stock for 25 minutes or until al dente.
2. Bring a pan of very salty water to a boil. Have a bowl with ice water handy. Place the peas in the boiling water for a minute. Remove and place immediately in the ice water.
3. Follow the same procedure for the broccoli, but cook for approximately 2 minutes or until al dente.
4. Place 1 Tbsp olive oil in a nonstick pan over medium heat. Add the butternut squash and cook until golden brown. Remove from pan and allow to cool.
5. In a separate bowl, add the ginger, 1 Tbsp olive oil, ½ of the parsley, the tea, and the peach juice. Blend with a hand blender. Refrigerate.
6. Place the barley, corn, butternut squash, peas, broccoli, and cucumber in a bowl with the greens.
7. Add the dressing, toss, and salt to taste.
8. To serve, place on a plate and sprinkle with the remaining parsley.

***Notes*** • *It is important to wash the greens to remove grit and dirt. Drain and pat dry, or use a salad spinner.* • *Chilling the peas and broccoli florets in ice water immediately after cooking preserves their beautiful bright green color.* • *You may substitute apple juice for peach, but peach is better.*

*Serves 4*
***Nutritional information per serving***
Calories 278
Protein 12g
Carbohydrates 48g
Fat 6g

# Vegetarian Sweet Potato and Lentil Salad

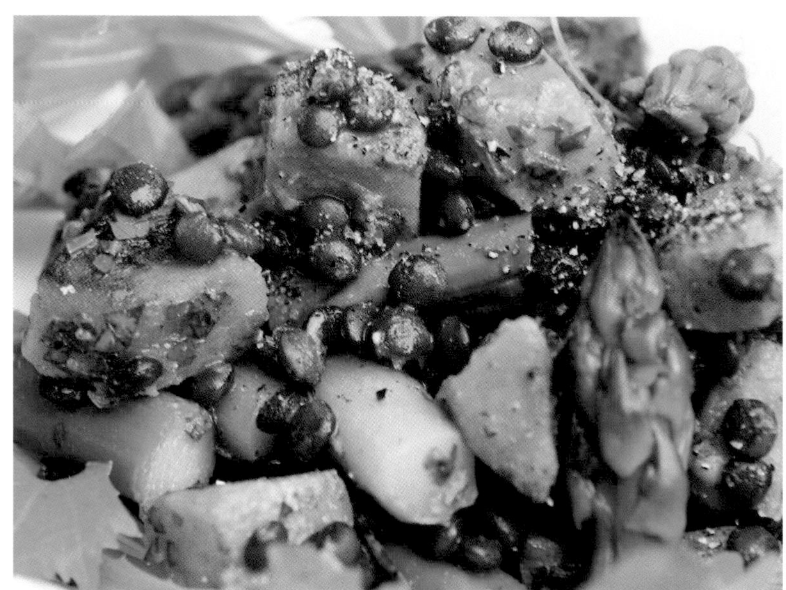

## Ingredients

- 1½ lbs (5 cups) sweet potato (peeled and cut into ½-inch pieces)
- 1 Tbsp olive oil
- ½ cup lentils
- 3 cups vegetable stock
- 2 Tbsp Roquefort cheese
- ½ tsp cardamom
- 8 oz (2 cups) asparagus (peel the bottom 3 inches of the stem, cut into 1-inch pieces)
- ¼ cup fresh parsley (washed, stems removed, chopped coarse)
- 1 Tbsp fresh thyme (washed, stems removed, chopped fine)
- 2 Tbsp fresh oregano (washed, stems removed, chopped fine)

## Directions

1. Cook the lentils in 3 cups of vegetable stock for about 45 minutes or until tender.
2. Cook asparagus in boiling salted water until tender. Place immediately in ice-cold water. Drain.
3. Sauté the sweet potatoes in a nonstick pan with the olive oil.
4. Drain the lentils, and mix in a bowl with the Roquefort cheese and ground cardamom.
5. Add the lentils, parsley, thyme, oregano, and asparagus to the potatoes.
6. Serve immediately.

***Notes*** • *When cooking dry lentils, do not add salt until the very end. Otherwise, the beans will not be tender.* • *This salad can be served warm in the winter or cold in the summer.* • *Canned lentils can be substituted. Rinse well and drain before adding to the potatoes.* • *Asparagus stems are very tough and fibrous, which is why it is best to peel the bottom 3 inches or just discard them.*

# Asian Tuna Tartare

*Serves 4*
*Nutritional information per serving*
Calories 285
Protein 27g
Carbohydrates 6g
Fat 16g

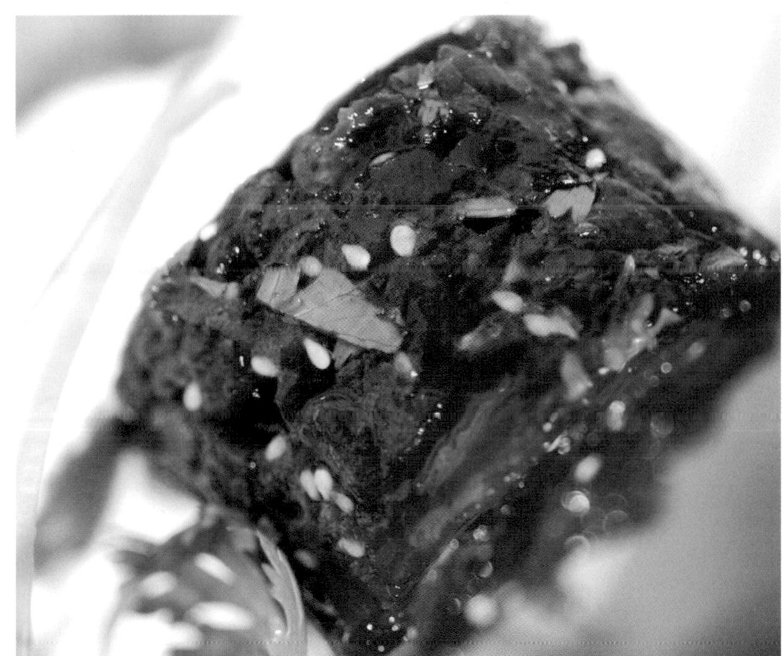

### Ingredients

2 tsp ginger (peeled and grated fine)
2 Tbsp extra-virgin olive oil
1 lb sushi-quality tuna
½ tsp sesame seeds (toasted until golden brown)
2 tsp fresh lemon rind (grated fine)
4 Tbsp soy sauce
15 sprigs cilantro (washed, stems removed, and chopped fine)
Salt to taste
1 Tbsp carrot (peeled and chopped fine or grated)
8 thin croutons (oven dried until light golden brown)

### Special equipment

Round mold or open-ended cookie cutter, 2¼ inches in diameter and 1½ inches high

### Directions

1. Trim silver skin from the tuna. Cut into tiny cubes (no bigger than ⅛ inch). Put the tuna in a mixing bowl. The recipe to this point can be made up to five hours ahead; cover and refrigerate.
2. Forty-five minutes or less before serving, add 1 Tbsp olive oil along with the sesame seeds, lemon rind, soy sauce, ginger, and cilantro to the tuna. Mix gently. Season with salt. Fill the mold with the tuna tartare mixture, pressing it gently so the tuna is even and compact. Place the mold upside down in the center of the salad plate. Remove the mold. Repeat, making 3 more plates.
3. Drizzle the remaining oil on the plates around the tartare. Sprinkle the carrot over the oil. Serve with the croutons.
4. Optional: Serve pita bread or thin, fresh slices of baguette on the side.

***Notes*** • *The carrots are used for garnish and color. Another option is to use sprigs of cilantro or microgreens.*

# Prosciutto-Wrapped Asparagus Crêpes

*Serves 6*
*Nutritional information per serving*
Calories 123
Protein 8g
Carbohydrates 15g
Fat 3g

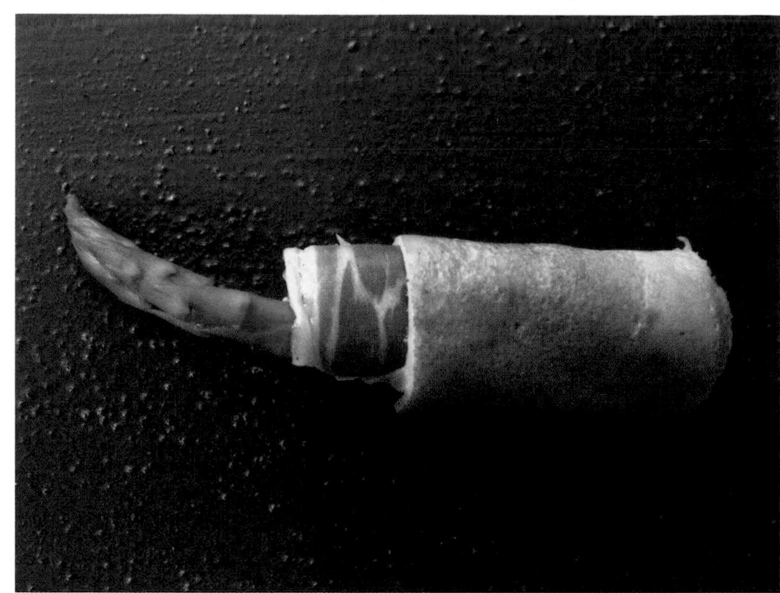

### Ingredients for the crêpes

¾ cup flour
1¼ cups (10 fl oz) milk
2 eggs
Nonstick spray
1 Tbsp Parmesan cheese

### Ingredients for the crêpe filling

½ lb jumbo asparagus
3 slices prosciutto (with the white layer of fat and skin removed)

### Directions for the crêpes

1. Place the flour in a large bowl.
2. With a whisk, make a well in the middle of the flour to create room for the eggs and milk. Add ⅓ of the milk, and whisk in a small circle in the middle of the bowl until it is a thick paste.
3. Avoid touching the side of the bowl with the whisk. This could cause the flour to mix in too quickly, which will make the batter lumpy.
4. When the batter looks like thick pancake batter, add another ⅓ of the milk. Whisk until you achieve a thinner pancake batter. There should be no lumps.
5. Add the last ⅓ of the milk, and whisk until smooth. If you still have lumps, strain the batter through a fine strainer.
6. Add the grated Parmesan cheese. Whisk to combine.

### Directions for the filling

1. Cut 2 inches off the bottom of the asparagus.
2. Bring a large pot of water to a boil and add salt to make the water as salty as seawater.
3. Put the asparagus in the boiling water and cook until al dente.
4. Remove the asparagus, place in ice-cold water, and then drain.
5. Cut in half crosswise into approximately 4-inch pieces.

### Cooking the crêpe

1. Heat an 8-inch nonstick pan over medium low heat.
2. Spray with nonstick spray and wipe off the excess with a paper towel.
3. Add about 2 oz of the crêpe batter and swirl the batter over the whole pan. The layer of batter should be very thin, with no excess batter in the pan.
4. Cook until the bottom of the crêpe becomes golden brown. If it browns too fast, lower the temperature.
5. Flip with a spatula and cook for another 30 seconds.
6. Place the crêpe onto a plate and repeat the same procedure until the batter is used up.

### To serve

1. Cut the prosciutto slices in half lengthwise.
2. Place two pieces of asparagus on a piece of prosciutto and roll up. Place this in the middle of the crêpe. Fold the ends of the crêpe toward the middle, then roll up like a burrito.
3. Repeat until the asparagus and crêpes are used up.

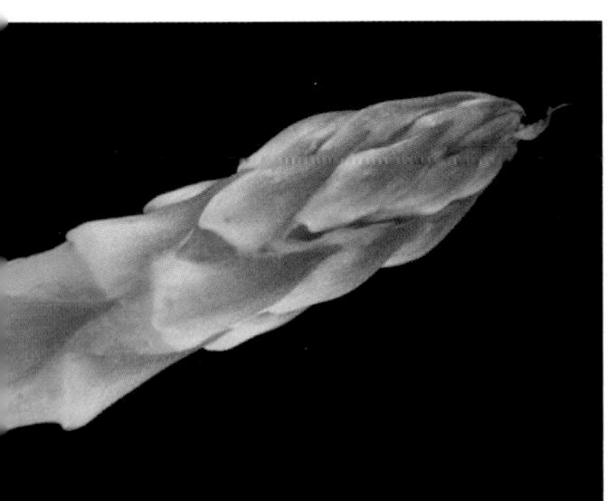

***Notes*** • *Shocking the asparagus in ice-cold water will help retain their bright green color.* • *Placing salt in the asparagus water seasons the asparagus and enhances its flavor.* • *To prevent the crêpes from getting too thick, pour any excess batter from the pan.* • *The asparagus, prosciutto, and crêpes can be assembled up to 5 hours before serving. Keep covered with plastic wrap.*

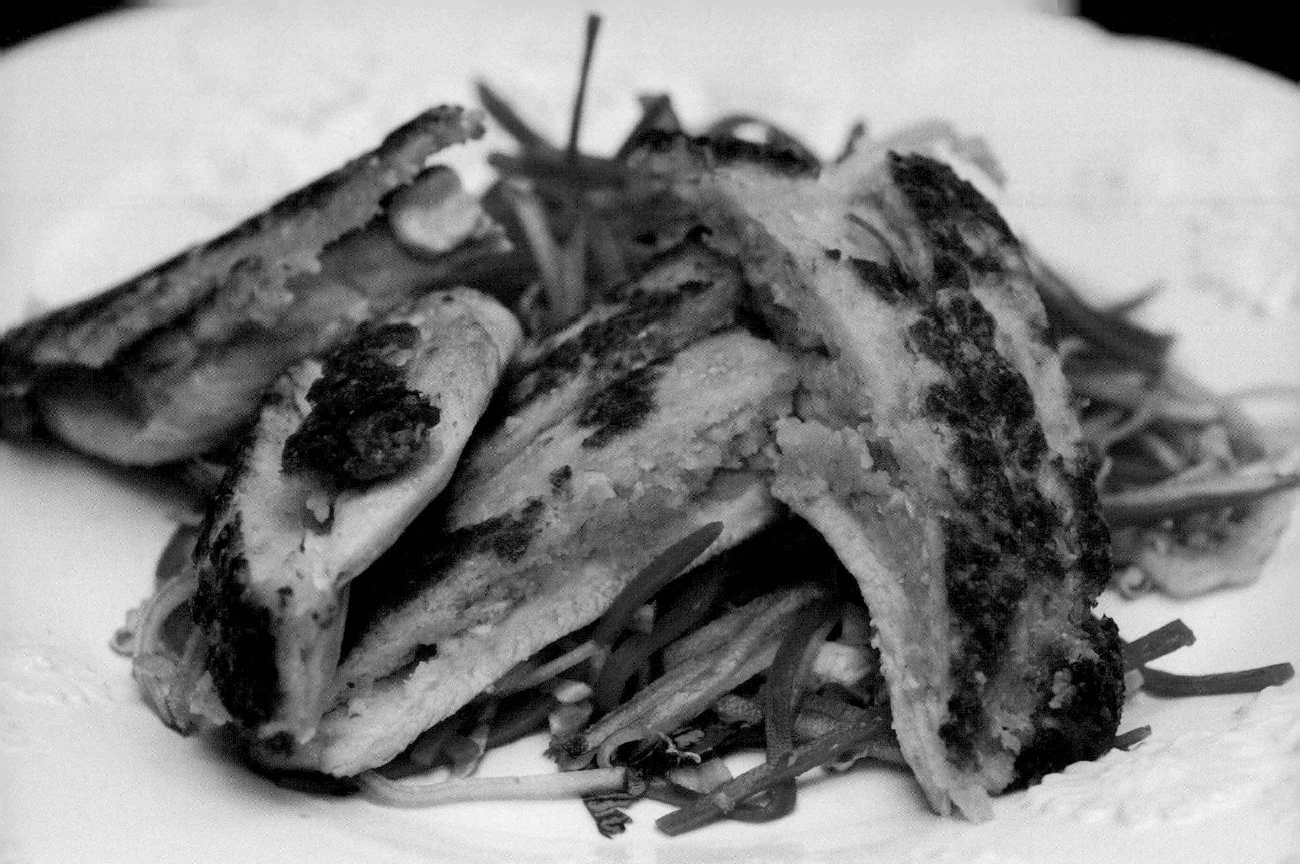

*Serves 4*
*Nutritional information per serving*
Calories 504
Protein 37g
Carbohydrates 46g
Fat 18g

# Crisp Asian Chicken Salad

## Directions for the chicken

1. Place the panko, oatmeal, and Parmesan cheese in a food processor. Gently process.
2. Butterfly each chicken breast by placing a knife along the side of the breast and sliding the blade horizontally to create ⅓-inch-thick cutlets. If the thickness is uneven, use a meat tenderizer to achieve even thickness.
3. Store on a paper towel, cover with plastic wrap, and refrigerate.
4. Break the eggs into a small bowl and add salt. Mix well with a fork for 1–2 minutes, and refrigerate.
5. To prepare the dressing, mix the brown sugar, soy sauce, plum sauce, and olive oil in a bowl.

### Ingredients for the chicken

- 4 chicken breasts (boneless, skinless)
- 1 cup panko (Japanese bread crumbs)
- ¼ cup oatmeal
- 2 Tbsp Parmesan cheese
- 2 eggs
- Salt to taste
- 2 Tbsp olive oil

### Ingredients for the salad

- 2 cups carrots (peeled and cut into long thin strips or grated)
- 2 cups Napa cabbage (washed, drained, and cut into thin strips)
- 1 cucumber (washed, peeled, cut into 2-inch pieces, then cut into thin strips or grated)
- ½ cup cilantro (washed, dried, stems removed, and chopped coarse)
- 1 ripe pear (washed, peeled, cut into thin strips or grated)

### Ingredients for the dressing

- 1 Tbsp brown sugar
- 1 Tbsp soy sauce
- 2 Tbsp plum sauce (or hoisin sauce)
- 1 Tbsp olive oil

### To serve

1. Dust the chicken breast on one side with flour.
2. Dip the floured side in the egg mixture, then the breadcrumb mixture.
3. Heat a nonstick pan over medium heat. Add 1 tsp of oil.
4. Place the breaded side of the chicken down in the pan. It should sizzle as it reaches the pan. Lower the temperature and cook until the breaded side is golden brown in color, approximately 2–3 minutes.
5. Flip and cook another 30 seconds just to coagulate the meat on the other side.
6. Let rest 2–3 minutes.
7. In a bowl, mix the carrots, Napa cabbage, cucumber, cilantro, and pear.
8. Add the dressing to taste and mix.
9. Add salt, as needed.
10. Place the salad on a plate.
11. Cut the cooked chicken breast into thin strips and place atop the salad.

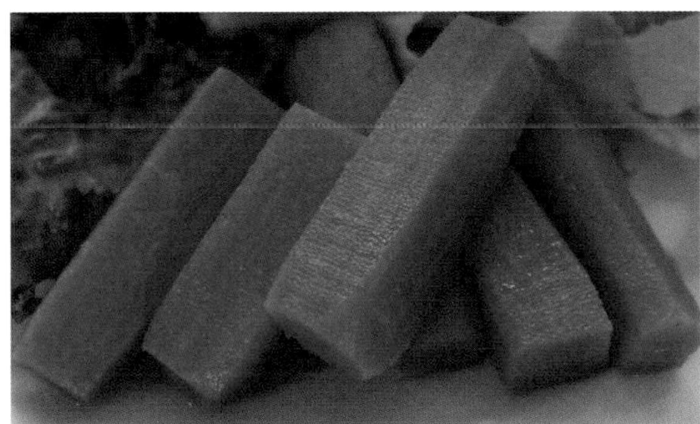

***Notes*** • *Julienning is the French term for cutting food into small "matchsticks." Ideally, they should each be 2 inches long and ⅛-inch thick.* • *Dipping the breast in flour before dipping in the breadcrumb mixture helps the breadcrumbs stick to the breast. I like to dip only one side of the breast, as I cook the breast mostly on the side with the breadcrumbs. Otherwise, it overcooks and dries out.*

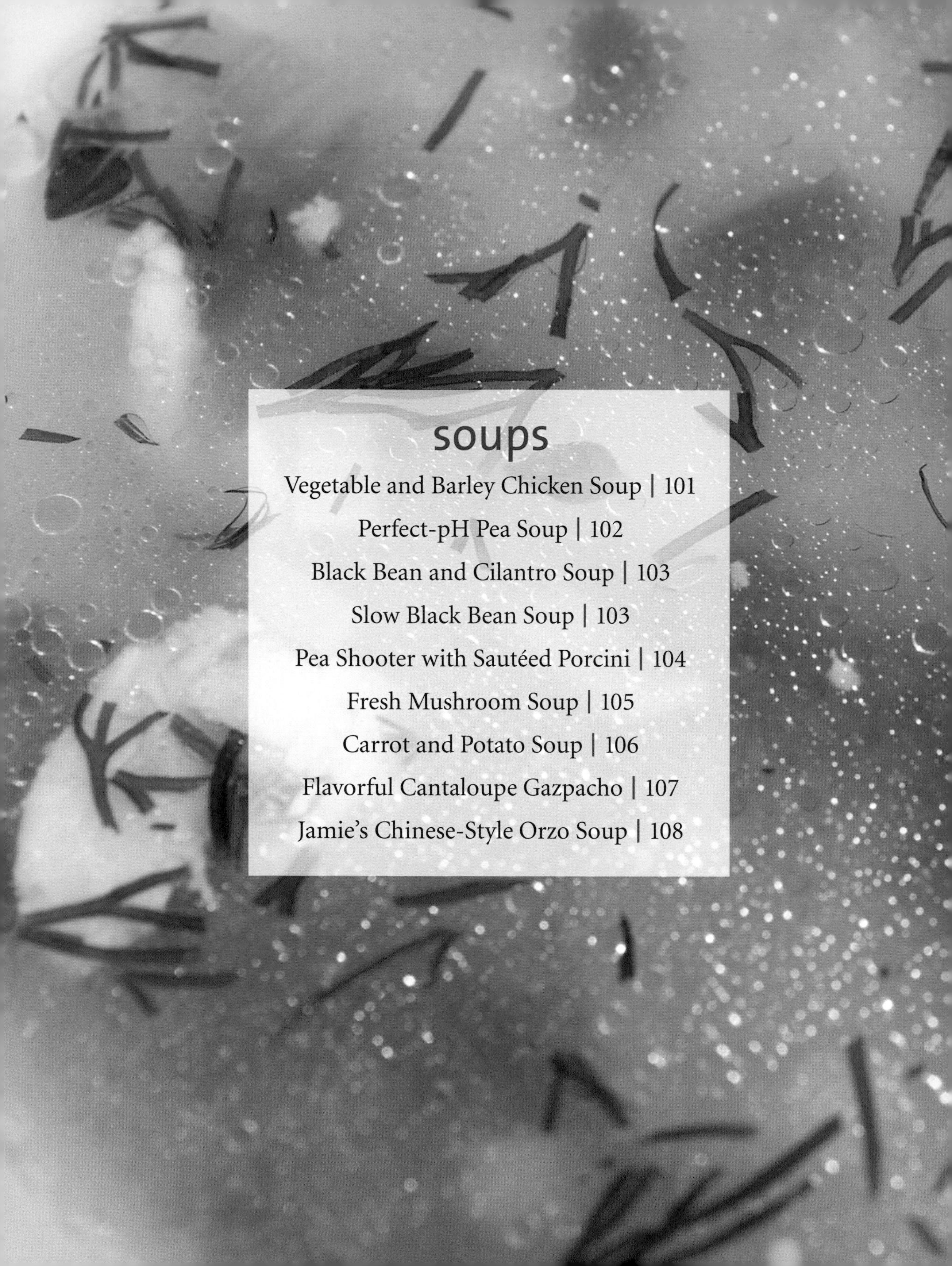

# soups


Vegetable and Barley Chicken Soup | 101

Perfect-pH Pea Soup | 102

Black Bean and Cilantro Soup | 103

Slow Black Bean Soup | 103

Pea Shooter with Sautéed Porcini | 104

Fresh Mushroom Soup | 105

Carrot and Potato Soup | 106

Flavorful Cantaloupe Gazpacho | 107

Jamie's Chinese-Style Orzo Soup | 108

*Serves 12*
***Nutritional information per serving***
Calories 194
Protein 25g
Carbohydrates 14g
Fat 4g

# Vegetable and Barley Chicken Soup

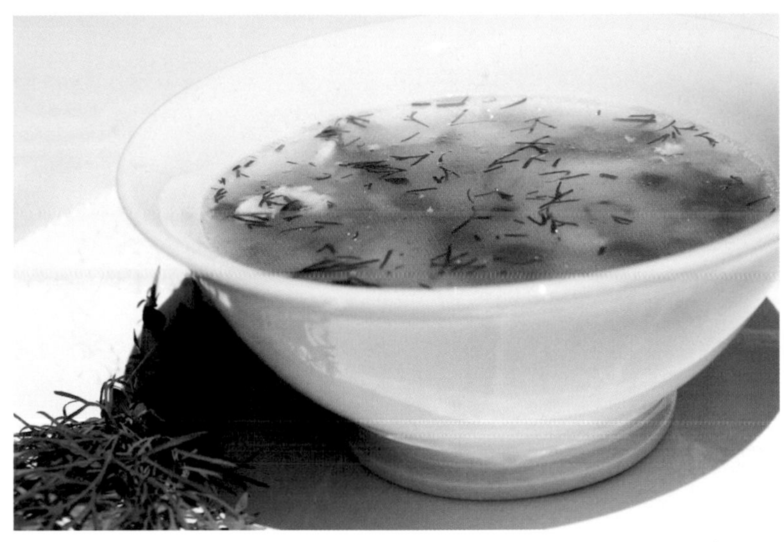

## Ingredients

1 chicken (approx 3 lbs, skin and wing tips removed, cut into 4 pieces or left whole)
2 cups carrots (peeled, washed, cut into ¼-inch pieces)
1 Idaho potato (about ¾ lb, peeled and cut into ¼-inch pieces)
1 cup barley
10 sprigs dill (optional)
4 bay leaves
10 sprigs thyme (washed and tied together with butcher's twine)
1 stalk celery (washed and cut into ⅓-inch pieces)
1 cup parsnip (peeled and cut into ¼-inch pieces)
1 Tbsp salt

## Directions

1. Place the chicken in a large pot with the carrots, potato, barley, dill, bay leaves, thyme, celery, and parsnips.
2. Cover with water at least 1½ inches above the chicken.
3. Bring to a boil and cook slowly for about 45 minutes to 1 hour.
4. Remove the chicken and place on a cutting board.
5. Once cool, remove all bones and cut or shred the meat into bite-size pieces.
6. Place the boneless pieces of chicken back into the soup.
7. Add more stock or water, as needed, as some of the liquid may have evaporated during cooking.
8. Add salt, as needed.
9. Serve immediately or cool to room temperature and refrigerate for up to 5 days.

**Notes** • *This soup freezes well. After it reaches room temperature, pour into freezer containers and place deep inside the freezer.*

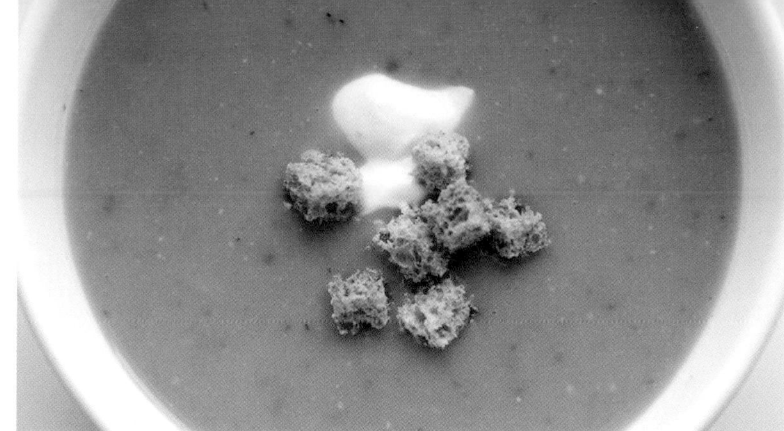

# Perfect-pH Pea Soup

***Serves 6***
***Nutritional information per serving***
Calories 310
Protein 22g
Carbohydrates 52g
Fat 3g

## Ingredients

- 1 lb split peas (soaked in the refrigerator overnight in cold water)
- 2 quarts chicken stock
- 2 oz (4 slices) prosciutto (fat removed, cut into small strips)
- 3 sprigs thyme
- 2 bay leaves
- 1 tsp salt (or more, as needed)
- 2 Tbsp nonfat sour cream
- 3 slices white bread (crust removed, cut into ¼-inch pieces)

## Directions

1. In a medium saucepan, place the drained peas, prosciutto, and chicken stock. Bring to a simmer.
2. Wrap the thyme and bay leaves with butcher's twine and attach to the handle of the pot for easy removal. Cook for about 45 minutes.
3. Remove the thyme and bay leaves.
4. Use a hand blender, regular blender, or food mill to blend the soup to a silky-smooth texture.
5. Add salt to taste. (Normally very little is needed because the prosciutto is quite salty.)
6. Serve or cool for later use.
7. Preheat oven to 325°F. Place the cubes of bread (croutons) on a cookie sheet and put in the oven until golden brown. Keep at room temperature until needed.

## To serve

1. Reheat the soup, stirring frequently with a wooden spoon.
2. Adjust consistency with chicken stock, as needed.
3. Serve in a soup bowl, garnished with the croutons and 1 tsp nonfat sour cream.
4. You can run a skewer through the sour cream to create an attractive design on the surface of the soup.

**Notes** • *If you don't have time to soak the split peas, blanching them in hot water will work as well. Do not add salt to the peas yet, as it interferes with the softening of the peas and slows down the cooking process. (The same applies to all beans.)* • *If you do not cook the split peas on a low simmer, the soup may burn on the bottom of the pot.* • *I like to cook the croutons in a very low-temperature oven (300–325°F) to lower the risk of burning them.* • *The soup tends to thicken as it sits on the stove. Add chicken stock to adjust the consistency.* • *Caution: The soup can scorch easily during reheating because of its starchy consistency.* • *There is almost no fat in this recipe, because we first trim the fat from the prosciutto.* • *Thyme and bay leaves are called a Bouquet Garni because they look like a little bouquet of herbs.*

# Black Bean and Cilantro Soup

***Serves 3***
***Nutritional information per serving***
Calories 72
Protein 4g
Carbohydrates 11g
Fat 1g

### Ingredients

8 oz canned black beans (drained and rinsed with clear water)
1 pint chicken stock
½ cup fresh cilantro (washed, roots removed, and chopped with the stems)
Salt to taste
1 Tbsp nonfat sour cream (for garnish)

### Directions

1. In a medium saucepan, bring the chicken stock to a boil. Add the beans, cilantro, and salt.
2. Cook 30 minutes on low heat.
3. Blend with a hand blender to the desired consistency.
4. Season, as needed.
5. Serve in a soup bowl and garnish with 1 tsp nonfat sour cream and a sprig of cilantro.

***Notes*** • *The cilantro stems give the soup a great flavor.* • *Add more chicken stock if the soup is too thick.*

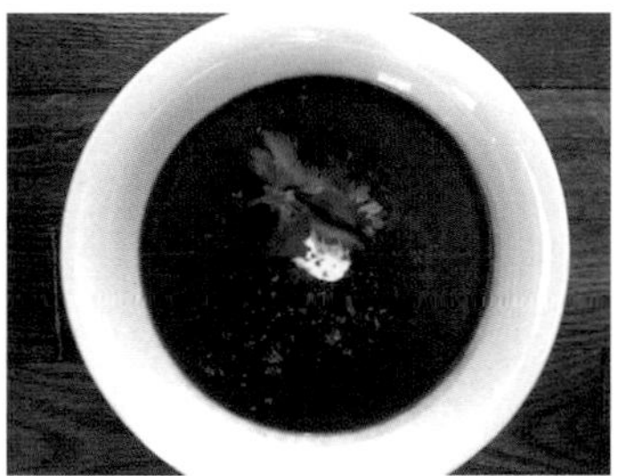

# Slow Black Bean Soup (Using Dried Beans)

***Serves 6***
***Nutritional information per serving***
Calories 261
Protein 17g
Carbohydrates 48g
Fat 1g

### Ingredients

1 lb dry beans (covered with cold water for 1 hour, then drained)
2 quarts chicken stock
1 cup fresh cilantro (washed, roots removed, and chopped with the stems)
Salt to taste
Nonfat sour cream (for garnish)

### Directions

1. Bring the chicken stock to a boil.
2. Add the beans and cilantro.
3. Cook 90 minutes on low heat.
4. Blend with a hand blender to the desired consistency.
5. Season, as needed.
6. Serve in a bowl and garnish with a spoonful of nonfat sour cream and a sprig of cilantro.

***Notes*** • *The cilantro stems give the soup a great flavor.* • *This soup needs double the cooking time of the pea soup recipe (opposite) because of the dry beans.* • *Do not add the salt at the beginning, or the beans won't cook properly.* • *Add chicken stock if the soup is too thick.* • *You can add lean smoked meat for a smoky flavor.*

# Pea Shooter with Sautéed Porcini

*Serves 10*
***Nutritional information per serving***
Calories 96
Protein 5g
Carbohydrates 12g
Fat 3g

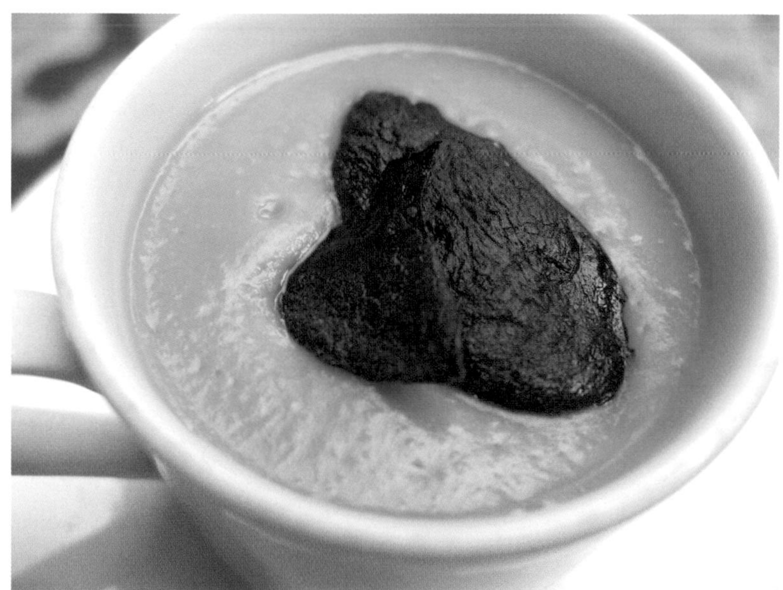

### Ingredients for the pea soup

1 lb (3 cups) baby peas (if not available, use regular size)
1 pt chicken stock
6 Tbsp whole milk
1 Tbsp brown sugar

### Ingredients for the porcini topping

½ cup dried porcini (soaked for 10 minutes in warm water, drained)
2 Tbsp butter

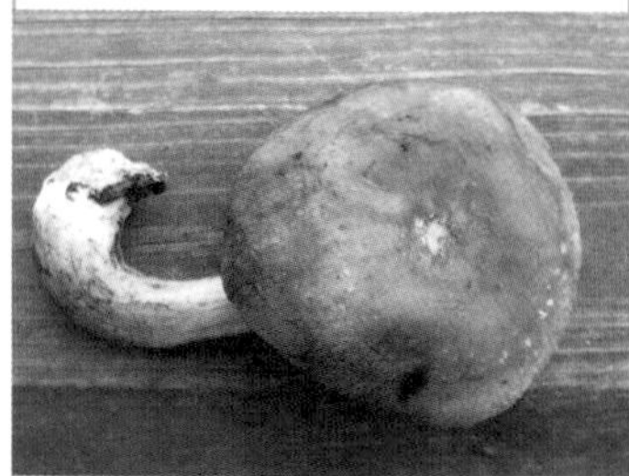

### Directions for the pea soup

1. Bring the chicken stock to a boil.
2. Add the peas and brown sugar, then simmer for about 15 minutes.
3. Place in a blender for about a minute, and add milk until the desired consistency is reached.
4. Season, as needed.

### Directions for the porcini topping and for serving

1. Heat a small pan over low heat. Add the butter and porcini mushrooms. Cook for about 2 minutes, until seared. Add salt.
2. Cut into small pieces, approximately ¼ inch.
3. Serve soup either hot or cold in small shooter glasses.
4. Sprinkle the top with the porcini mushrooms.
5. Serve immediately.

**Notes** • *This is a delicious soup to have as the first course of a dinner. It can be served hot during the winter and cold during the summer.*

# Fresh Mushroom Soup

***Serves 6***
***Nutritional information per serving***
Calories 63
Protein 6g
Carbohydrates 14g
Fat 1g

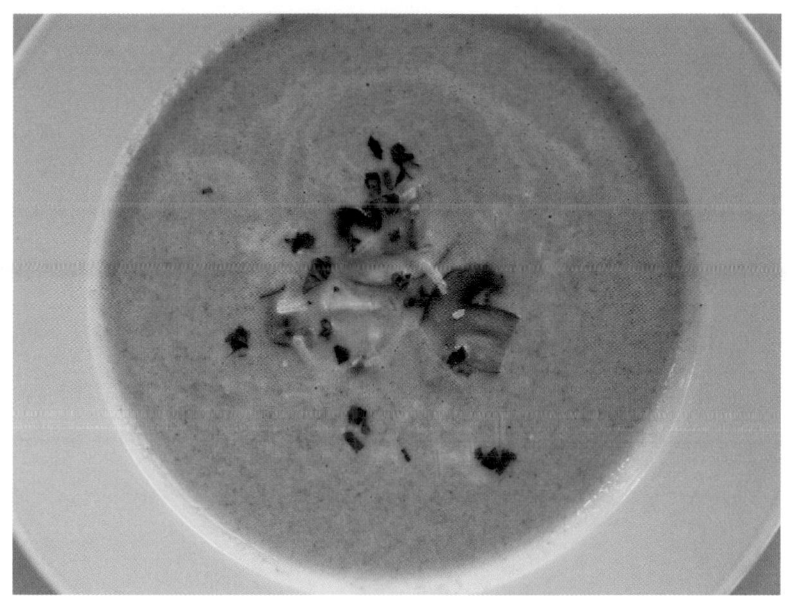

## Ingredients

1 lb domestic mushrooms
½ qt whole milk
½ qt chicken stock
2 bay leaves
3 sprigs thyme
Salt to taste
2 tsp Parmesan cheese, grated
4 sprigs flat-leaf parsley (stems removed, chopped fine and dried in a paper towel)
2 slices white bread (optional: crusts removed)

## Directions

1. Wash mushrooms 2–3 times by lifting them from a bowl filled with cold water. Proceed until the water is clear. (Mushrooms often have sand in them.)
2. Remove about ¼ inch from the bottom of the mushroom stem, cut in half lengthwise, and cut as thin as possible.
3. Place the milk, stock, thyme, and bay leaves in a saucepan and bring to a simmer. Add the mushrooms and cook for about 40 minutes.
4. Remove the thyme and bay leaves. Using a high-speed blender, blend the soup to a smooth consistency.
5. Add salt to taste.
6. Place the soup into a bowl, and sprinkle with grated Parmesan cheese and chopped parsley.

***Notes*** • *Do not pour the water from the bowl after washing the mushrooms, as some of the dirt will reattach to the mushrooms. The best way to wash mushrooms is to have two bowls. Fill one with water, add the mushrooms, and agitate. Lift the mushrooms and place in the empty bowl. Then fill the second bowl with water and do the same until the mushrooms are clean.* • *Using a high-speed blender allows the soup to get velvety without adding any cream or fat. A hand blender will also work, but the consistency won't be as smooth.* • *If the soup is too thin, blend one or two slices of white bread (crust removed) with the finished soup. The starch from the bread will slightly thicken it.* • *If you like a deeper taste to the soup, you can add about 1 Tbsp dried mushrooms.* • *You can also garnish the mushroom soup with sautéed sliced mushrooms that have been caramelized in a tablespoon of olive oil or butter. The caramelized (brown-colored) mushrooms add a great earthy taste.*

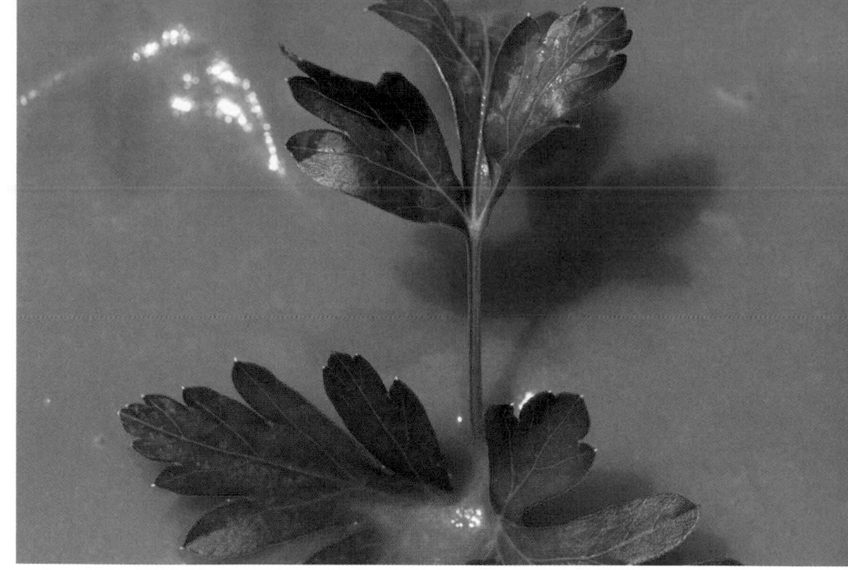

# Carrot and Potato Soup

***Serves 4***
***Nutritional information per serving***
Calories 64
Protein 1g
Carbohydrates 14g
Fat 1g

## Ingredients

1 lb carrots (peeled, diced into ½-inch cubes)
12 oz (2½ cups) Idaho potatoes (peeled and diced into 1-inch cubes)
1 qt chicken stock
1 Tbsp fresh ginger (peeled and cut into ¼-inch pieces)
1 Tbsp fresh parsley (washed, stems removed, cut into fine strips, dried on a paper towel)

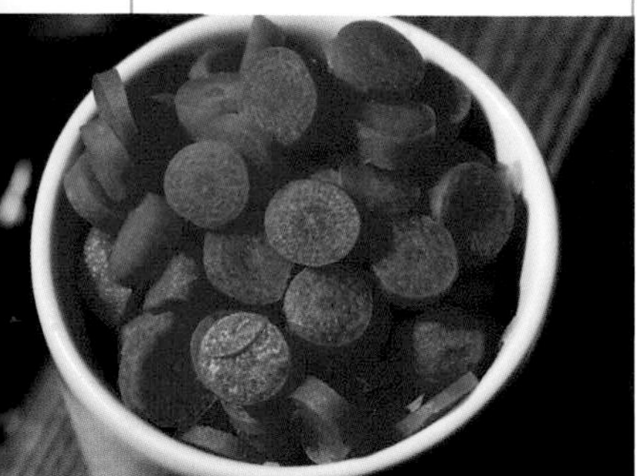

## Directions

1. Place the carrots, potatoes, chicken stock, and ginger in a large saucepan. Simmer for about 40 minutes on low heat.
2. Place the soup in a blender and blend until smooth. Season as needed.
3. Serve in a bowl and garnish with the parsley.

**Notes** • *If the soup becomes too thick, add chicken stock.*

*Serves 2*
***Nutritional information per serving***
Calories 180
Protein 2g
Carbohydrates 41g
Fat 1g

# Flavorful Cantaloupe Gazpacho

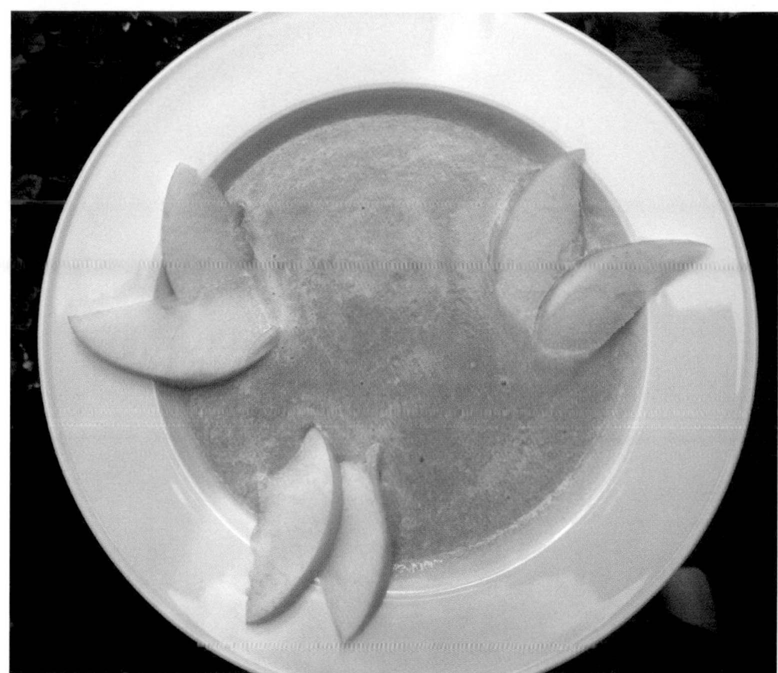

## Ingredients

1 lb (2 cups) cantaloupe (skin removed, seeded, cut into 1-inch pieces)
3 Tbsp brown sugar or agave sugar
2 Tbsp port wine
Dusting of finely grated nutmeg

## Directions

1. Mix the cantaloupe, sugar, and port. Place in the freezer for about 4 hours.
2. Blend in a blender.
3. Finish with a dusting of nutmeg.
4. Serve immediately in a shot glass or small cup.

***Notes*** • *This is a refreshing summer soup. If using as a dessert, add more ice when blending.* • *You can use honeydew for this recipe as well, but use white port instead so that the soup maintains a light yellow-green color.*

# Jamie's Chinese-Style Orzo Soup

*Serves 14*
*Nutritional information per serving*
Calories 64
Protein 1g
Carbohydrates 14g
Fat 1g

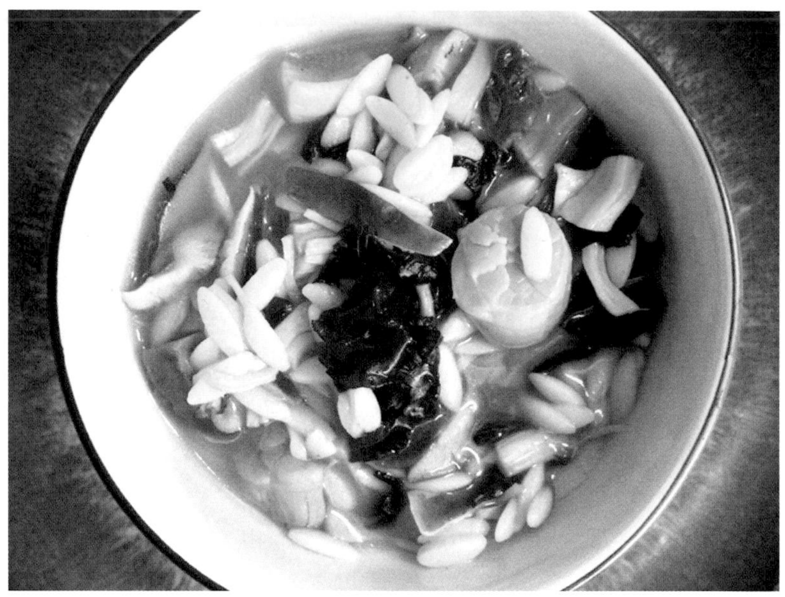

## Ingredients

- 1 (4 oz) package sliced shitake mushrooms
- 1 (4 oz) package Cremini mushrooms (use the smaller ones and quarter them)
- 3 chicken stock bouillon cubes (vegetable if you are vegetarian)
- 10 cups water
- 1 Tbsp soy sauce
- ½ small box Chinese black fungus (auricula), rehydrated (makes 1½ cups) chopped coarse
- 1 cup dried scallops
- 1 cup orzo
- 1–2 tsp sea salt
- ½ cup fresh cilantro (optional)
- 1 medium bunch of fresh spinach (optional)

## Directions

1. On the morning of making the soup (or the night before), place the dried scallops and black fungus in a large bowl and add hot water. After a few minutes, dump out the water and add fresh hot water. This helps remove some of the salt.
2. That evening, drain the scallops and fungus. Chop the fungus coarse.
3. Combine all the ingredients except for the orzo and salt, and bring to a boil uncovered.
4. Simmer 30 minutes, then add the orzo and salt to taste.
5. Bring to a gentle boil, stirring frequently; simmer another 20–30 minutes.
6. Add spinach and/or cilantro at the end.
7. Serve in cups or bowls with a spoon.

***Notes*** • *One of the pleasures of living in New York is that I can shop Chinatown for special ingredients that make delicious one-pot meals.* • *I usually make this dish on Friday evenings so I can enjoy it all weekend.* • *I prefer North Sea scallops, because they are large and reasonably priced. I usually buy a pound at a time to make 2–3 pots of soup.* • *I also love the black fungus, also called "auricular." It is uniquely chewy/crunchy with little taste but a wonderful texture.* • *Orzo is a pasta shape that's like gigantic soft rice when cooked. It can turn a simple soup into a satisfying one-pot meal.* • *Dishes like this combine great flavors and textures and contain almost no fat.* • *Sometimes, I add fresh spinach, cilantro, and/or meat such as turkey breast cut into small cubes.*

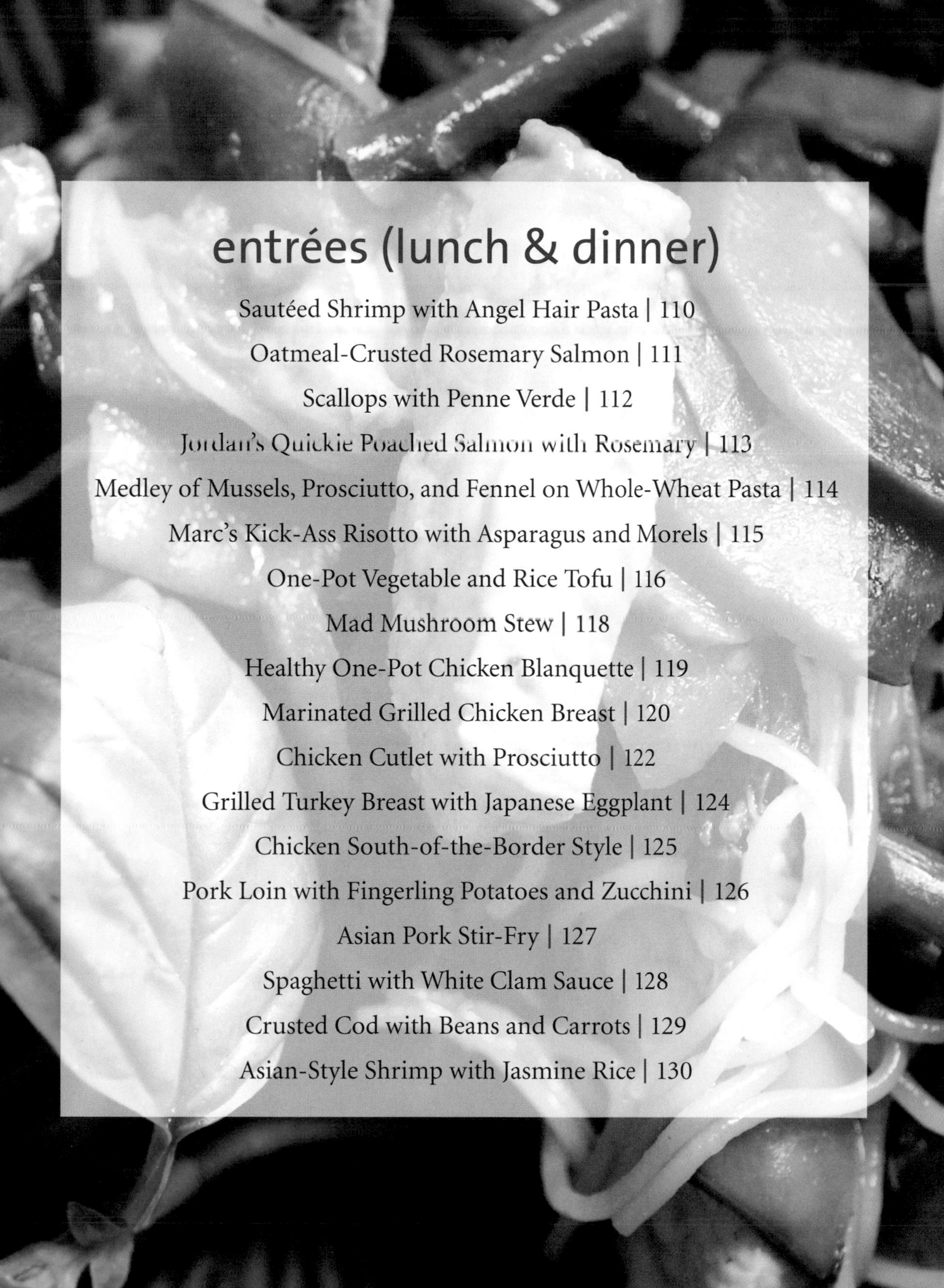

# entrées (lunch & dinner)


Sautéed Shrimp with Angel Hair Pasta | 110

Oatmeal-Crusted Rosemary Salmon | 111

Scallops with Penne Verde | 112

Jordan's Quickie Poached Salmon with Rosemary | 113

Medley of Mussels, Prosciutto, and Fennel on Whole-Wheat Pasta | 114

Marc's Kick-Ass Risotto with Asparagus and Morels | 115

One-Pot Vegetable and Rice Tofu | 116

Mad Mushroom Stew | 118

Healthy One-Pot Chicken Blanquette | 119

Marinated Grilled Chicken Breast | 120

Chicken Cutlet with Prosciutto | 122

Grilled Turkey Breast with Japanese Eggplant | 124

Chicken South-of-the-Border Style | 125

Pork Loin with Fingerling Potatoes and Zucchini | 126

Asian Pork Stir-Fry | 127

Spaghetti with White Clam Sauce | 128

Crusted Cod with Beans and Carrots | 129

Asian-Style Shrimp with Jasmine Rice | 130

# Sautéed Shrimp with Angel Hair Pasta

*Serves 4*
***Nutritional information per serving***
Calories 578
Protein 34g
Carbohydrates 84g
Fat 13g

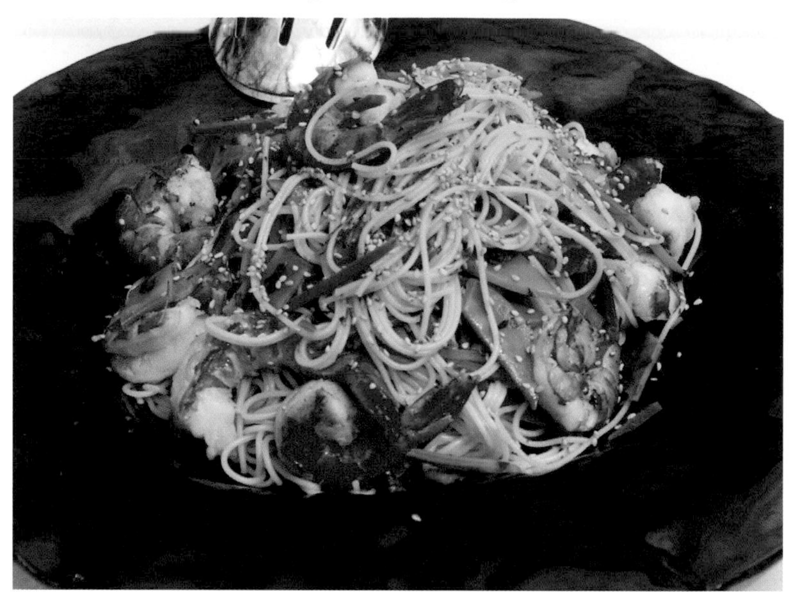

## Ingredients

- 1 lb shrimp (16 to 20 shrimps per lb, shelled and deveined)
- ¾ lb angel hair pasta (capellini)
- 1 lb snow peas (tips removed, cut into 1-inch diamond shape by cutting on the bias)
- 1 cup carrots (peeled and grated or cut on a mandoline to make long, thin sticks)
- 1 cup chicken stock
- 1 (8 oz) bottle clam juice
- 5 sprigs thyme (washed, stems removed, chopped fine)
- ½ cup parsley (washed, stems removed, chopped fine)
- 2 tsp sesame seeds (toasted to an amber color)
- 2 Tbsp extra-virgin olive oil

## Directions

1. Fill a large pot with water and bring to a boil. Add salt.
2. Add the pasta and cook for about 3–4 minutes. Drain.
3. Heat a nonstick pan with 1 Tbsp of the olive oil. Sear the shrimp until the flesh is opaque on both sides, approximately 4–6 minutes. Remove the shrimp and keep warm.
4. Drain the excess oil and add the second tablespoon of oil to the pan. Sear the snow peas and carrots for about 1 minute.
5. Add clam juice, chicken stock, thyme, parsley, and half of the sesame seeds, and bring to a simmer.
6. Add the pasta and shrimp, and toss. Add salt as needed.
7. Serve in a soup bowl or deep dish, and sprinkle with the remaining sesame seeds.
8. Garnish with a few shrimp and a sprig of thyme.

***Notes*** • *It is important to cook the shrimp just until the flesh turns opaque. Otherwise, it loses most of its natural water and becomes chewy.* • *I use olive oil, as it adds a nice flavor. I leave some of the oil in the pan when I add the clam broth.*

*Serves 4*
***Nutritional information per serving***
Calories 431
Protein 50g
Carbohydrates 6g
Fat 21g

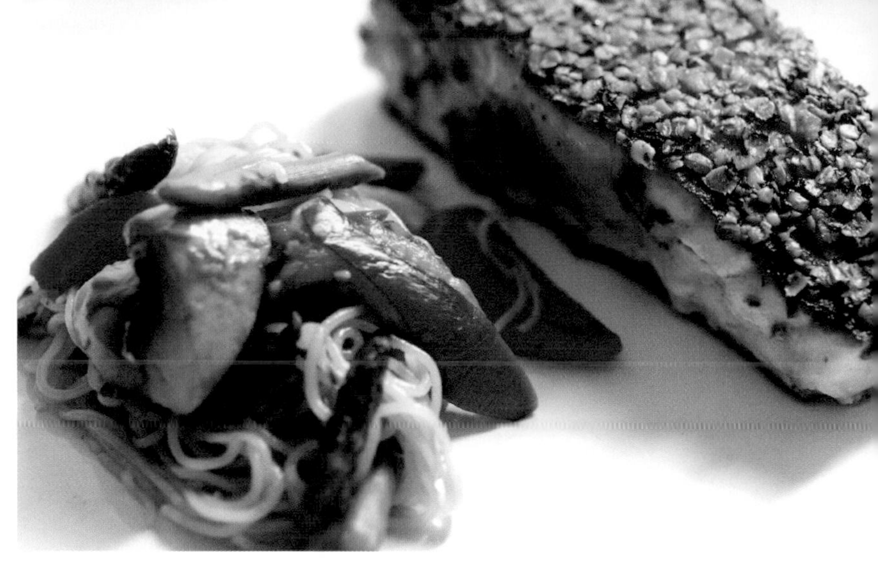

# Oatmeal-Crusted Rosemary Salmon

## Ingredients

- 2 lbs salmon filet (trimmed, skinless, pin bones removed, cut into 8-oz portions)
- 1 tsp lemon zest
- 1 Tbsp white miso paste
- 10 sprigs rosemary (stems removed, chopped fine)
- 5 Tbsp dry oatmeal
- 1 Tbsp canola oil

## Directions

1. In a small bowl, mix the lemon zest, miso paste, and rosemary.
2. Brush it over the salmon and let sit in the refrigerator, covered, for 5 minutes or up to 2 hours.

## To serve

1. Remove the salmon from refrigerator.
2. Dip the presentation side (usually the side with the pin bones) into the oatmeal, which will adhere to the miso-lemon mix.
3. Heat a large nonstick pan over medium heat.
4. Add the oil and, when sizzling, add the salmon. Lower the temperature slightly and cook until the oatmeal turns golden brown, approximately 5–7 minutes.
5. Flip with a wide nonstick spatula and cook another 5 minutes.
6. Drain on a paper towel to remove excess fat.
7. Serve over a salad or with a vegetable of your choice.

***Notes*** • *Salmon can be replaced with sablefish, arctic char, or scallops.* • *If the salmon is from a reputable fish market, you can maintain its moist texture by cooking just until the center is slightly translucent.* • *The miso paste, rosemary, and lemon zest provide the flavor. The canola oil has not been flavored, so we remove it by resting the salmon on two paper towels.* • *Make sure you dip the salmon in the oatmeal right before cooking, or the oatmeal will get soggy.* • *Overcooking salmon (or any fish) dries it out.*

*Serves 4*
***Nutritional information per serving***
Calories 514
Protein 38g
Carbohydrates 82g
Fat 4g

### Ingredients for the scallops

1 lb or 12 large sea scallops (remove the tough little muscle on the side)
2 Tbsp olive oil

### Ingredients for the Verde sauce

2 cups chicken stock
2 cups basil (stems removed, tightly packed, washed 3 times or until no sand remains)
3 Tbsp Parmesan cheese (grated)
1 cup cooked cannellini beans (or 1 cup canned white beans, drained)

### Ingredients for the pasta

¾ lb penne pasta (Barilla or DeCecco)

# Scallops with Penne Verde

### Directions for the Verde sauce

1. In a blender, add the basil and 1 cup chicken stock.
2. When it's smooth, add the beans and the Parmesan cheese.
3. Blend again until smooth.
4. Reserve in a sealed container.

### Directions for the pasta

1. Bring a pot of water to a boil and add salt.
2. Place the pasta in the boiling water and cook until al dente, about 7–10 minutes. Drain and reserve.

### To serve

1. Pat the scallops dry with a paper towel. Season with salt.
2. Heat a sauté pan over medium heat and add the olive oil.
3. Add the scallops carefully. The oil should sizzle loudly without smoking or flaring up. Cook on medium for about 3 minutes or until the scallops turn golden brown.
4. Flip and cook another 3 minutes or so. Adjust heat as needed.
5. Remove and drain on a paper towel. Keep in a warm place.
6. Drain the oil from the pan.
7. Add 1 cup of the chicken stock to deglaze the pan and loosen the scallop juices.
8. Add the Verde sauce to taste, then the pasta. Bring to a simmer. Season with more salt if needed.
9. Serve the pasta in a soup bowl with the scallops on top.

***Notes*** • *The size of the scallops is not important, but be careful. Smaller scallops cook much faster, so adjust cooking time accordingly.* • *Only 10 percent of the cooking oil is counted toward the total of calories, as most of it is discarded after cooking.* • *Scallops should not smell like the sea! They should have a sweet neutral smell. Use them fresh or flash frozen; it makes a huge difference to the taste of the dish.* • *The foot of the scallop is the little protrusion sometimes present on the side. It is actually a muscle to hold the scallop to the shell.* • *If you don't have time to cook cannellini beans or northern beans in chicken stock for two hours with thyme and bay leaf, drain a small can of cannellini beans and rinse first before using.* • *The basil will be bright green for only a short time, so prepare it just before you need it. The oxidation of the chlorophyll turns it a darker green as it sits in the refrigerator.* • *I like to make a large batch of pesto and freeze it in small portions so that it is available quickly.*

# Jordan's Quickie Poached Salmon with Rosemary

***Serves 4***
***Nutritional information per serving***
Calories 514
Protein 38g
Carbohydrates 82g
Fat 4g

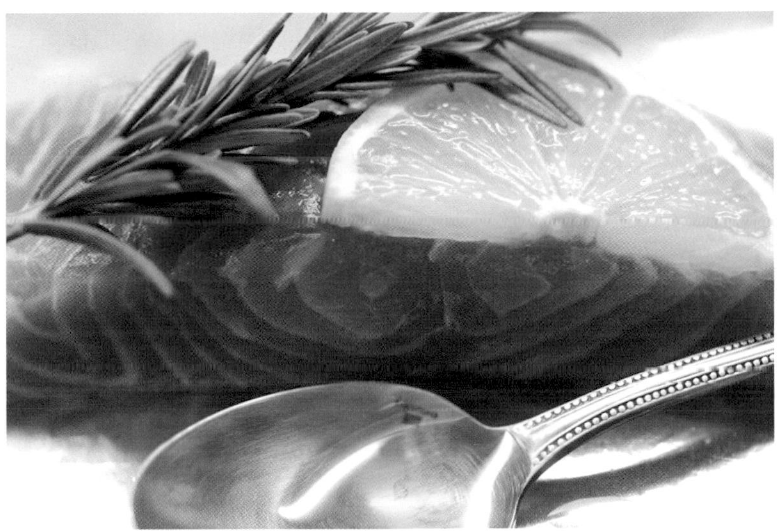

### Ingredients

4 salmon filets, 4 oz apiece
4 sprigs fresh rosemary
4 half-slices fresh lemon
1 tsp olive oil

### Directions

1. Place each filet skin-side down on a sheet of aluminum foil large enough to wrap the entire filet.
2. Place lemon and rosemary on the filet and drizzle ¼ tsp of the olive oil. Season with salt as needed.
3. Wrap each filet in foil and place in a baking pan in the oven at 350°F for 10–15 minutes.
4. To serve: Remove from oven, unwrap foil, and remove the lemon (do not squeeze it on the filet) and the rosemary.
5. Serve with rice and your favorite steamed greens.

**Notes** • *Prep time is about 5 minutes for the salmon.* • *The tightly wrapped foil allows the filets to steam. The rosemary (or other herbs of your choice) and the slice of lemon impart great flavor.* • *Since you are not squeezing the lemon on the fish, you avoid its acidity while enjoying the flavor—especially from the lemon skin that steams along with the filets.* • *You can leave out the olive oil drizzle if you prefer.* • *For accompanying vegetables, I usually steam asparagus, broccoli, or spinach.*

# Medley of Mussels, Prosciutto, and Fennel on Whole-Wheat Pasta

***Serves 4***
***Nutritional information per serving***
Calories 430
Protein 32g
Carbohydrates 64g
Fat 7g

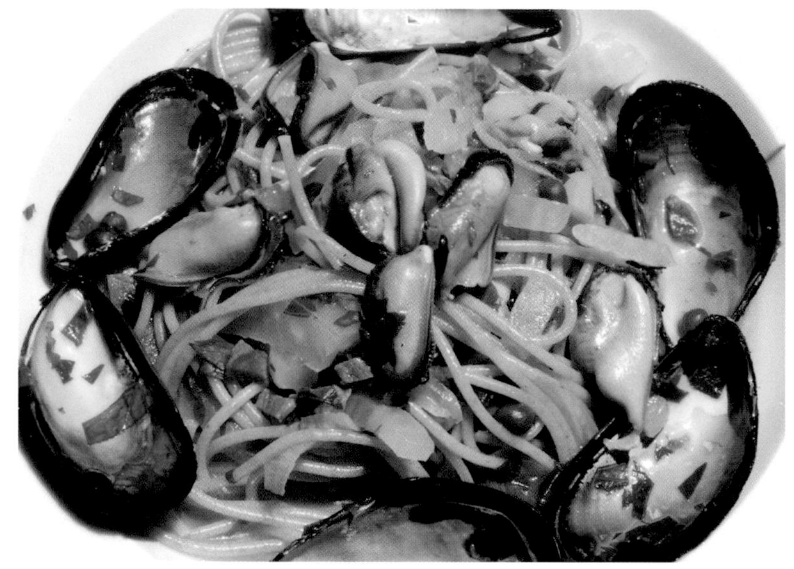

## Ingredients

- 1½ lbs mussels (washed and rinsed, beards removed from the shells)
- ½ fennel (julienned)
- 1 cup chicken stock
- 1 cup fresh parsley (washed, stems removed, chopped coarse and squeezed in a paper towel to remove excess chlorophyll)
- 2 Tbsp capers
- 2 oz (4 slices) prosciutto (excess skin and fat removed, cut into very thin strips, then diced)
- 12 oz thin spaghetti (preferably whole-wheat)
- 4 oz edamame (frozen, shells removed) (soy beans)

## Directions

1. Bring a large pot of water to a boil and add enough salt to taste like the sea.
2. Add the pasta and bring to a boil. Cook about 7 minutes and drain.
3. In a large pot, simmer the fennel, prosciutto, edamame, capers, and chicken stock about 4 minutes. Add the mussels to the chicken stock broth, cover, and cook about 5 minutes or until the mussels open fully.
4. Place the pasta in a large bowl. Pour the mussels and broth over it and mix thoroughly. Garnish with the parsley.
5. Serve in a soup bowl.

***Notes*** • *Prosciutto is one of the best flavorings and meats for* ***The Reflux Diet.*** *It has great taste and texture, and is reasonably low in fat once the fat is trimmed off. In this recipe we use only two ounces, which is about four slices trimmed and diced.* • *To julienne the fennel, cut lengthwise, place the flat side down on a cutting board, and cut across the fiber in very thin slices. A mandoline or a Japanese mandoline works well for slicing fennel thin.* • *If the mussel shells take up too much room on the plate, remove shells from half the mussels. It will be easier to handle and make the plate look more attractive.* • *I like Prince Edward Island (PEI) mussels because they're usually very clean.* • *Mussels go bad quickly. It is important to discard any open ones. If they close after tapping them a little, they're okay.* • *Edamame can be found in the frozen section of Asian grocery stores. If you can't find any, use one cup of frozen lima beans instead, but cook only two minutes.*

# Marc's Kick-Ass Risotto with Asparagus and Morels

***Serves 2 (3, if an appetizer)***
***Nutritional information per serving***
Calories 294 (196)
Protein 15g (10g)
Carbohydrates 58g (37g)
Fat 3g (2g)

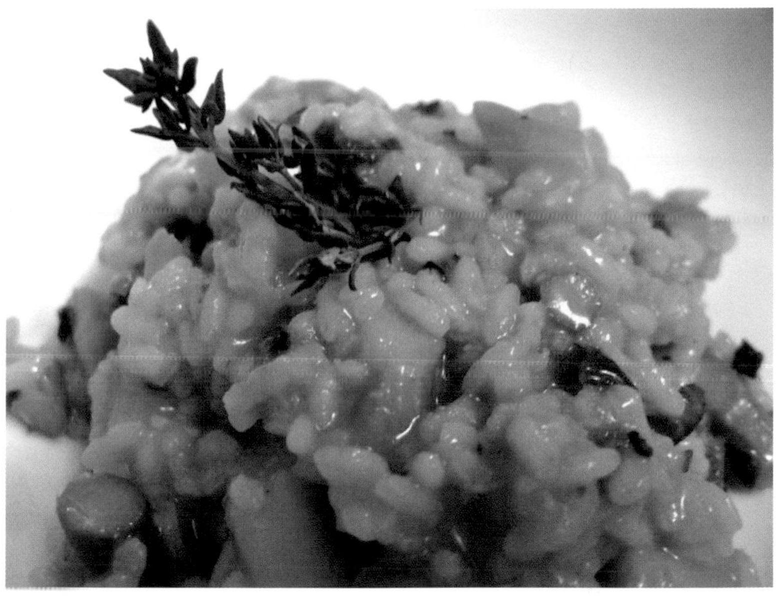

## Ingredients

1 cup arborio rice
1 bunch asparagus (about 1 lb) (peel the skin 3 inches below the head, cut to 1-inch lengths)
3 Tbsp dried morel or porcini mushrooms (soak for 1 hour in water or vegetable stock)
2 cups vegetable stock (or 1 vegetable bouillon cube dissolved in 2 cups water)
2 bay leaves
4 sprigs thyme
2 Tbsp Parmesan cheese
Salt to taste

## Directions

1. Remove the reconstituted mushrooms from the water. Reserve the liquid.
2. Bring the vegetable stock (or vegetable bouillon cube and water), thyme, bay leaf, and reserved mushroom liquid to a boil. Cook for 5 minutes and remove bay leaf and thyme.
3. Cook the asparagus in the stock for a few minutes until al dente. Remove and cool immediately to preserve the green color. Reserve the stock.
4. Place a saucepan over medium heat. Add the rice and ½ cup of the stock. Bring to a simmer while continuing to stir.
5. Once the rice has absorbed nearly all the liquid, add another ½ cup of the stock and continue to stir until the rice is creamy and al dente, about 20 minutes. Add more stock if the rice is too al dente or dry.
6. Add the asparagus, reconstituted mushrooms, and Parmesan cheese, and salt to taste. Serve immediately in a soup bowl.

***Notes*** • *Adding 2 tsp of Roquefort cheese to the risotto adds a twist to this classical dish.* • *The skin of the asparagus (about 3 to 4 inches below the head) tends to be fibrous. By peeling it, you'll get a nice al dente crunch. If dicing, cut on a bias.*

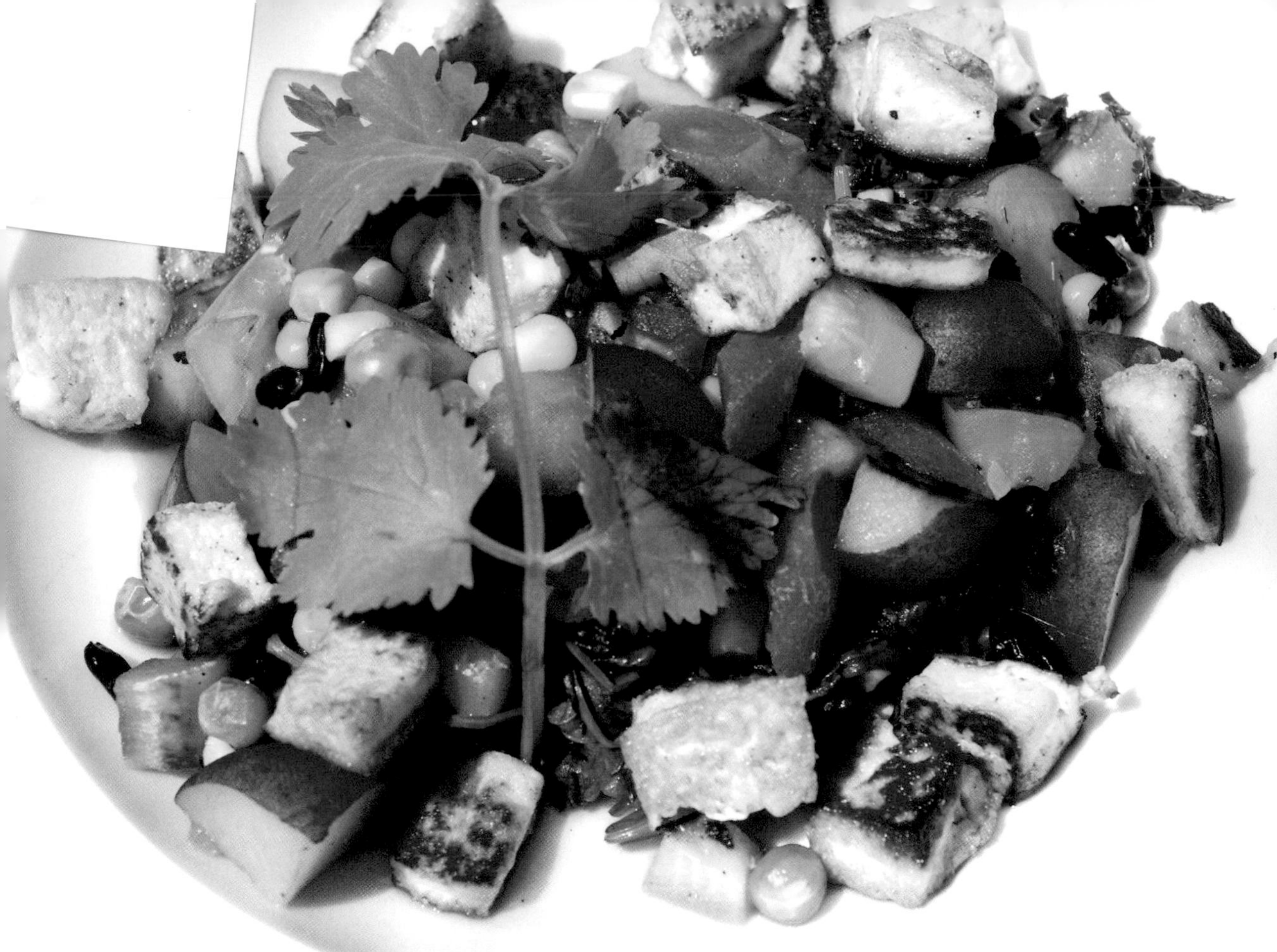

*Serves 6*
***Nutritional information per serving***
Calories 274
Protein 15g
Carbohydrates 47g
Fat 4g

# One-Pot Vegetable and Rice Tofu

### Directions for the rice

1. Bring the stock to a simmer. Add the rice, salt, stir, and cover.
2. Cook about 13 minutes on very low heat. Let rest another 10 minutes before serving.

### Directions for the vegetable tofu

1. Heat a nonstick pan with oil over medium heat. Add the tofu and sear until golden brown on one side.
2. Remove the tofu, and reserve. Drain excess fat from the pan with a ladle or drain.

### Ingredients for the rice

1 cup Japanese rice
1¼ cup vegetable stock
¼ tsp salt

### Ingredients for the vegetable tofu

1 lb extra-firm tofu (cut into ½-inch cubes and dried on paper towels)
1 Tbsp olive oil
½ cup carrots (peeled, trimmed, and cut into ½-inch sections on the bias)
1 cup red or fingerling potatoes (cut into ½-inch sections with the skin on)
½ cup zucchini (seeds removed, and diced into ½-inch cubes)
½ yellow squash (seeds removed, and diced into ½-inch cubes)
½ parsnip (peeled and diced into ½-inch cubes)
½ turnip (peeled and diced into ½-inch cubes)
½ stalk broccoli (cut into small florets)
½ cup peas
½ ear of corn (remove the corn with a knife or fork)
½ cup chicken stock
2 Tbsp soy sauce
½ cup Chinese fermented beans (soaked in cold water 5 minutes and drained)
1 cup fresh cilantro plus a few sprigs for garnish (tightly packed, washed, stems removed, chopped coarse)

### Directions for the vegetable tofu, cont.

3. Add the parsnips, turnip, carrots, potatoes, ¼ cup of chicken stock, and half the cilantro. Cook covered for 5 minutes.
4. Add the yellow squash, zucchini, broccoli, peas, corn, the remaining cilantro, soy sauce, fermented beans, and the remaining ¼ cup chicken stock.
5. Cook another 2 minutes, covered. Add the browned tofu, plus salt if needed, and serve immediately with the rice on the side.
6. Garnish with fresh cilantro.

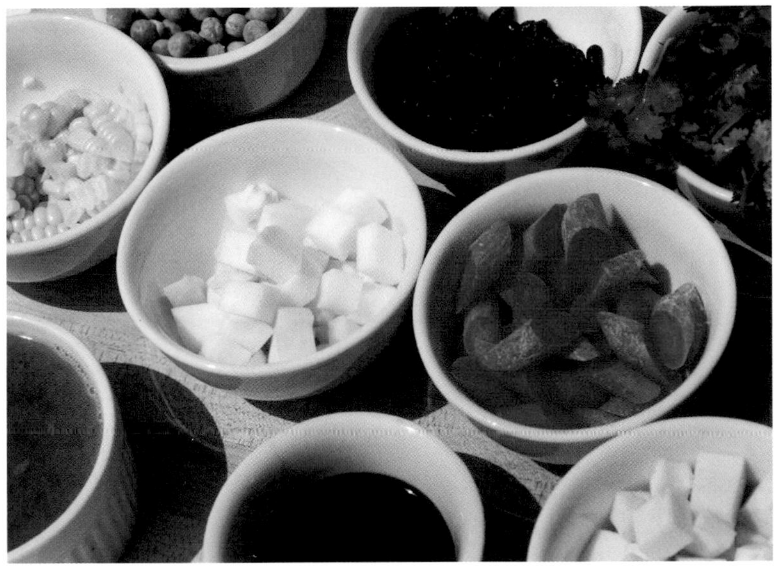

***Notes*** • *Make sure the lid fits tightly so the steam created by the stock and vegetables cooks the vegetables evenly.* • *It is important to dry the tofu on paper towels to remove excess water, or it will be difficult to achieve a golden-brown color.* • *The chopped cilantro brightens the dish's flavors.* • *You can find fermented beans in an Asian or Chinese grocery store.* • *Root vegetables take longer to cook and should be soft when done. The broccoli can be slightly crunchy.*

*Serves 5*
***Nutritional information per serving***
Calories 226
Protein 10g
Carbohydrates 34g
Fat 7g

# Mad Mushroom Stew

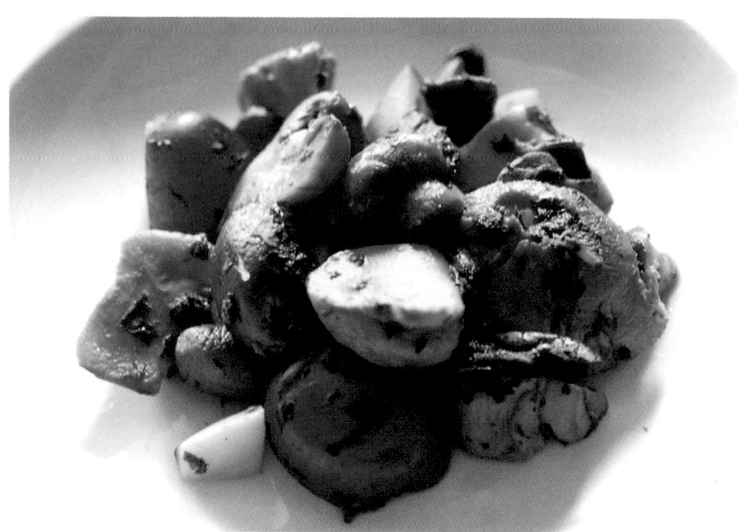

## Ingredients

- 8 oz (3 cups) cremini mushrooms
- 8 oz (3 cups) shitake mushrooms
- 1 lb (6 cups) domestic mushrooms (All of these fresh mushrooms should be washed, dried, ¼ inch trimmed from stem, and cut in quarters)
- 2 Tbsp olive oil
- ¼ cup dried porcini mushrooms (soaked in warm water 10 minutes, liquid reserved)
- 1 cup red potatoes (skin on, washed, diced into ½-inch cubes)
- 1 cup Yukon gold potatoes (skin on, washed, diced into ½-inch cubes)
- 1 cup parsnips (peeled, diced into ½-inch cubes)
- 1 Tbsp fresh parsley
- 1 Tbsp fresh rosemary
- 1 Tbsp fresh sage
- 1 Tbsp fresh thyme
- 1 cup chicken or vegetable stock
- 2 Tbsp grated Parmesan cheese
- 1½ tsp salt to taste

## Directions

1. Heat a sauté pan on high heat. Add the olive oil and sauté all mushrooms together.
2. When mushrooms are golden brown, add the potatoes, parsnip, parsley, rosemary, sage, thyme, and chicken stock. Bring to a boil, then lower heat to simmer. Cover. Potatoes will take 10–15 minutes to cook.
3. Place in a bowl or crock and sprinkle with the Parmesan cheese.
4. Serve immediately.

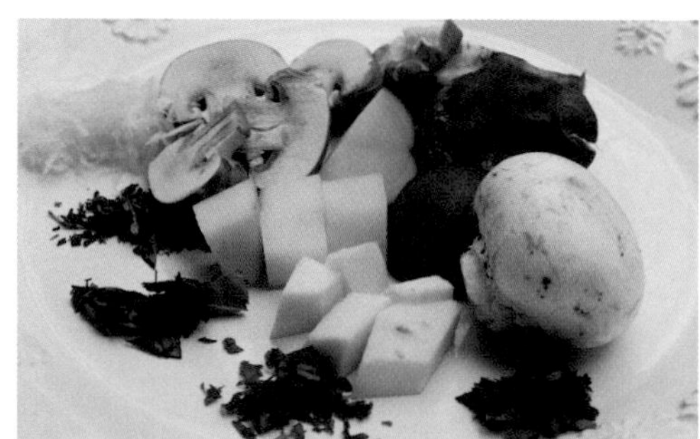

***Notes*** • *All of the fresh spices should have the stems removed and be chopped coarse.* • *Do not shake the pan excessively while cooking mushrooms, as they render water and start to boil instead of browning.* • *When cooking, if too much stock evaporates, add more as needed.* • *This is a great vegetarian dish if you use vegetable stock.*

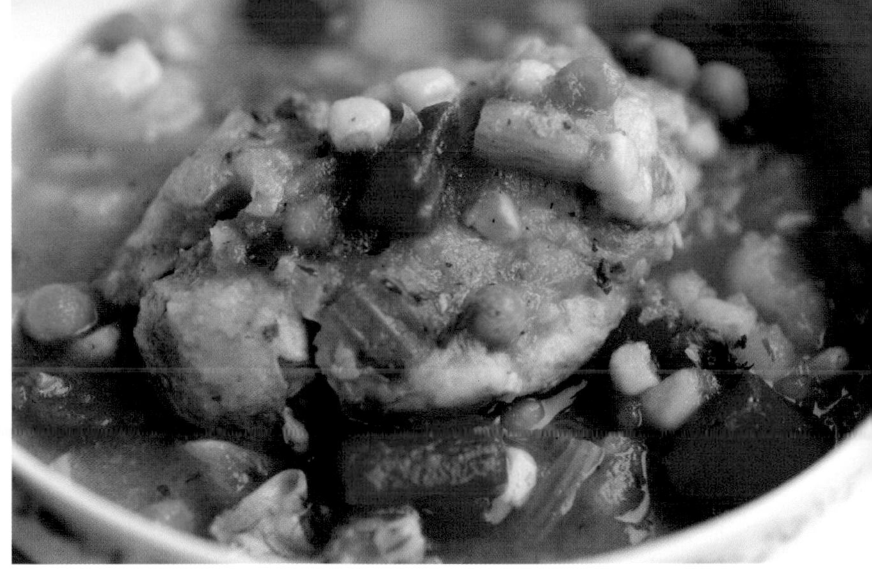

# Healthy One-Pot Chicken Blanquette (Stew)

***Serves 4***
***Nutritional information per serving***
Calories 295
Protein 21g
Carbohydrates 41g
Fat 4g

## Ingredients

4 chicken thighs (about 2 lbs)
1 cup carrots (peeled and diced into ½-inch cubes)
1 cup celery (peeled and diced into ½-inch cubes)
3 cups potato (peeled and diced into ½-inch cubes; keep in cold water to prevent oxidation)
4 cups chicken stock
1 cup frozen baby peas
1 cup frozen corn kernels (or fresh if preparing during summer or fall)
4 sprigs tarragon (stems removed, chopped fine)
4 sprigs parsley (stems removed, chopped fine)
½ cup oatmeal (or more if a thicker consistency is desired)
4 bay leaves
4 sprigs thyme
2 whole cloves (or ⅛ tsp ground)
1 dusting of nutmeg

## Directions

1. Remove the skin from the thighs and place in a large stockpot.
2. Add the celery, carrots, potato, and corn.
3. Cover with the chicken stock and bring to a boil.
4. Skim off the impurities that come to the surface.
5. Bring to a boil and skim*.
6. Add the bay leaves and thyme, which can be bundled with butcher's twine or in cheesecloth for easy removal after cooking.
7. Add salt to taste, then the nutmeg and cloves.
8. Simmer about 45 minutes. Add the rolled oats. If you use "instant," it will thicken faster.
9. Five minutes before serving, add the peas, tarragon, and parsley.
10. Serve in a crock or soup bowl.

*If you slowly bring the stew to a simmer, the liquid proteins (albumin) coagulate and float to the top of the broth.

**Notes** • *This is a hearty winter dish without the fat or onions. • You can use chicken breast or a whole chicken if you don't like thighs. The breast tends to dry out when cooked for an extended period. The thighs stay moist due to the "silverskin," or connective tissue, that turns into gelatin when cooked. • If you like the potato to have a little bite, use waxy potatoes (red or fingerling). I use Idaho potatoes, which also thicken the stew because of the starch content. • Notice that the green peas are added at the end. They take little cooking time and add an attractive color to the dish. Peas take under 5 minutes to cook. • Chopped tarragon and parsley are added to the stew just before serving to give it a fresh taste. • In France, the traditional Blanquette is made with veal.*

*Serves 4*
***Nutritional information per serving***
Calories 261
Protein 38g
Carbohydrates 28g
Fat 2g

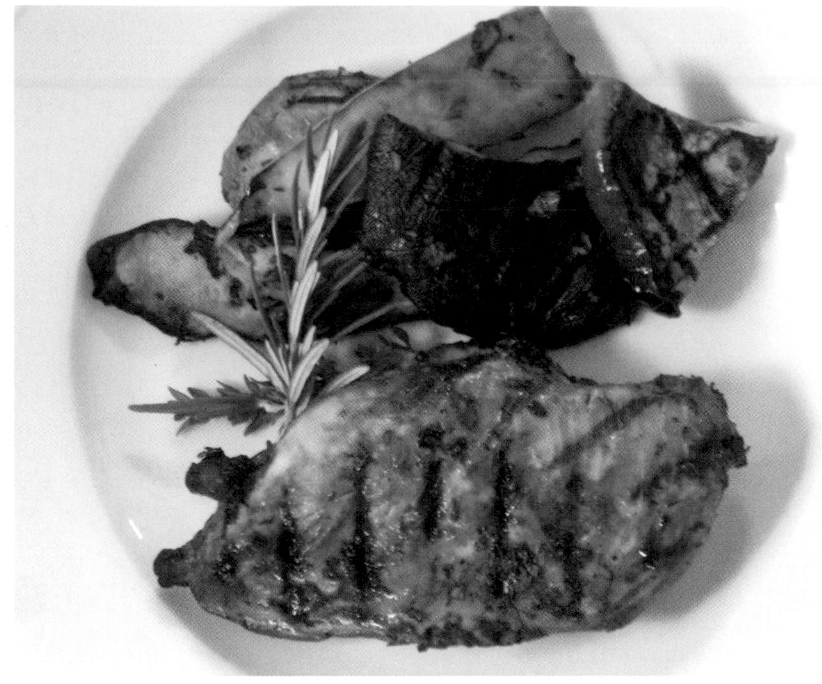

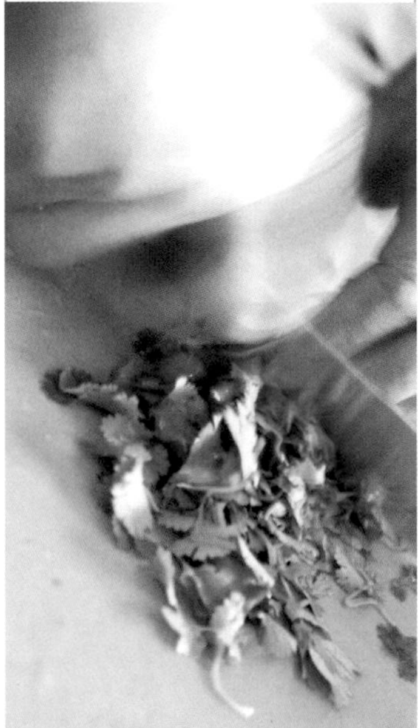

# Marinated Grilled Chicken Breast

### Directions for the chicken

1. In a bowl, whisk together the soy sauce, sugar, basil, thyme, rosemary, oil, and yogurt.
2. Place the chicken in a Ziploc bag and add half the marinade.
3. Seal the bag after removing excess air, and store in refrigerator.
4. Turn bag every hour to spread the marinade throughout the meat.
5. Marinate 2–12 hours.

### Directions for the grilled vegetables

1. Place the vegetable slices in a large Ziploc bag.
2. Add the other half of the marinade, remove excess air, seal and store in refrigerator.
3. Turn bag every hour to spread the marinade evenly.
4. Do not marinate more than 2 hours.

### Ingredients for the chicken

- 4 chicken breasts (skinless, boneless, tenderloin and fat removed)
- 1 cup soy sauce
- 1 Tbsp brown sugar
- 2 Tbsp fresh basil (washed, dried, leaves separated from the stems, chopped coarse)
- 2 Tbsp fresh thyme (washed, dried, leaves separated from the stems, chopped fine)
- 2 Tbsp fresh rosemary (washed, dried, leaves separated from the stems, chopped fine)
- 1 Tbsp oil
- ½ cup yogurt

### Ingredients for the grilled vegetables

- ½ lb (2 cups) zucchini (ends trimmed and cut on bias ¼-inch thick)
- ½ lb (2 cups) yellow squash (ends trimmed and cut on bias ¼-inch thick)
- ½ lb (3 cups) domestic mushrooms (washed, drained, and ¼ inch trimmed off the stem)
- ½ lb (2 cups) purple Sicilian eggplant (ends trimmed and cut on the bias about ¼-inch thick)
- 2 Tbsp oil for cleaning the grill (soak a rag lightly with the oil and wipe grill before using)

### To serve

1. Preheat grill or grill pan. Scrub grill with wire brush.
2. Soak a rag in a few drops of oil and wipe the brushed grill.
3. Remove the chicken breasts and vegetables from the bags.
4. Drain in a colander and pat dry with paper towels.
5. Place the chicken and vegetables on the grill, sear until golden brown, and flip.
6. Cook another few minutes until golden brown and flip again once or twice, making sure you get a diamond-shaped grill mark on at least one side of the chicken and vegetables.
7. If the chicken has a nice grill mark but is not completely cooked, finish in the oven or on a low-heat part of the grill.
8. Serve immediately on a plate. Display a variety of vegetables in a contrast of colors.

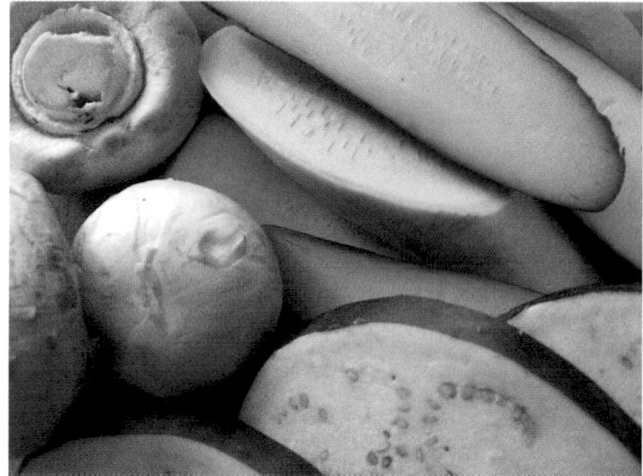

***Notes*** • *The rag will turn dark from the excess carbon left after brushing. The grill should smoke but not flare up; if it does, there was too much oil on the rag. Wipe again with another rag that has less oil.* • *Cutting ¼ to ½ inch off the mushrooms allows them to cook more evenly because they lie almost flat on the grill, giving them better exposure to the heat.* • *Because of the yogurt, the meat's tenderness increases if you let it marinate overnight.* • *You can also use this marinade with thin strips of skirt steak.* • *To avoid cross-contamination of bacteria, do not reuse the chicken marinade.* • *The amount of grilling time for the meat and vegetables depends on the temperature of the grill.*

# Chicken Cutlet with Prosciutto

***Serves 2***
***Nutritional information per serving***
Calories 267
Protein 26g
Carbohydrates 21
Fat 10g

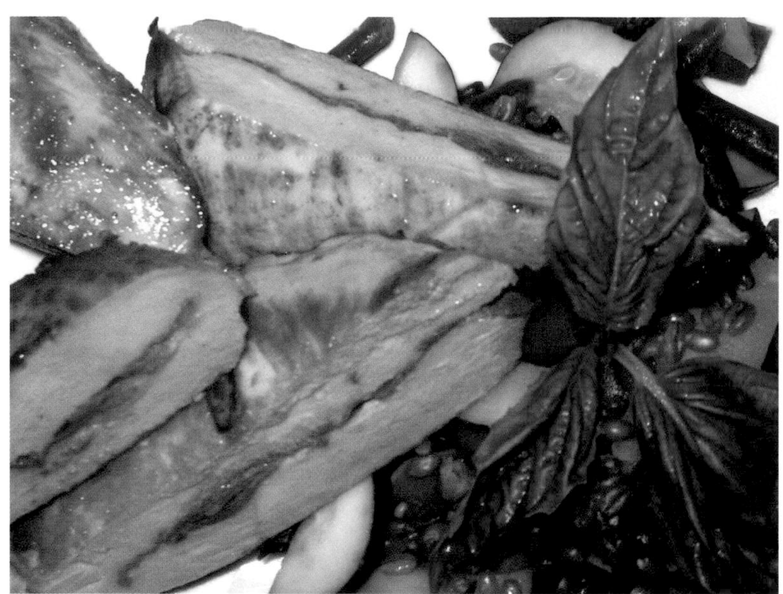

### Ingredients for the chicken

1 chicken breast, boneless, skinless (12 oz)
2 slices imported prosciutto, fat removed
2 Tbsp olive oil
1 garlic clove (peeled and cut in half so it can be removed from pan after the oil is flavored)

### Ingredients for the vegetables

1 cup zucchini (cut in half lengthwise and sliced thin to create half-moon shapes)
8 oz (2 cups) green beans (ends trimmed)
2 cups chicken stock (or more, if needed)
10 leaves fresh basil (washed, dried, leaves removed from stems, chopped fine)
1 cup parsnip (peeled, cut in half lengthwise and sliced thin)
½ cup carrots (peeled, diced into ⅓-inch cubes)
¾ cup barley
Salt to taste

### Directions for the chicken

1. Split the whole breast in half and place the two sides flat on a cutting board. Slice horizontally to yield two thin cutlets.
2. Place one thin slice of prosciutto over one of the cutlets, and cover with the second chicken cutlet so that the prosciutto forms a thin layer in the middle.
3. Repeat with the second half-breast.
4. With a meat pounder or the side of a chef's knife, gently pound the cutlet so it adheres to the prosciutto.
5. Cover and refrigerate until needed.

### Directions for the vegetables

1. In a medium pot, bring the chicken stock to a boil. Add the green beans and cook until al dente, about 7 minutes. Drain and reserve the stock.
2. Cook the zucchini (about 30 seconds), parsnip (3–4 minutes), and carrots (4–5 minutes) the same way as the beans. Drain and reserve the stock each time.
3. Cook the barley in the same stock (about 15–20 minutes). When the barley is al dente, drain and store until needed.

### To serve

1. In a nonstick pan over medium heat, add the 2 Tbsp olive oil and garlic. Cook until the garlic is golden brown.
2. Remove the garlic and immediately place the chicken breast in the same oil. Cook for about 2–3 minutes, then flip. Cook for another minute or two. When done, remove and reserve. Do not discard the oil.
3. In the same pan, add the zucchini, parsnips, carrots, green beans, and barley. Heat on medium.
4. If the vegetables seem dry, add chicken stock. The barley tends to absorb a lot of the liquid.
5. When the vegetables are warm, add salt as needed. Place the vegetables in a small mound on a plate. Cut the chicken cutlet in half lengthwise and place on top.
6. Garnish with chopped basil leaves.

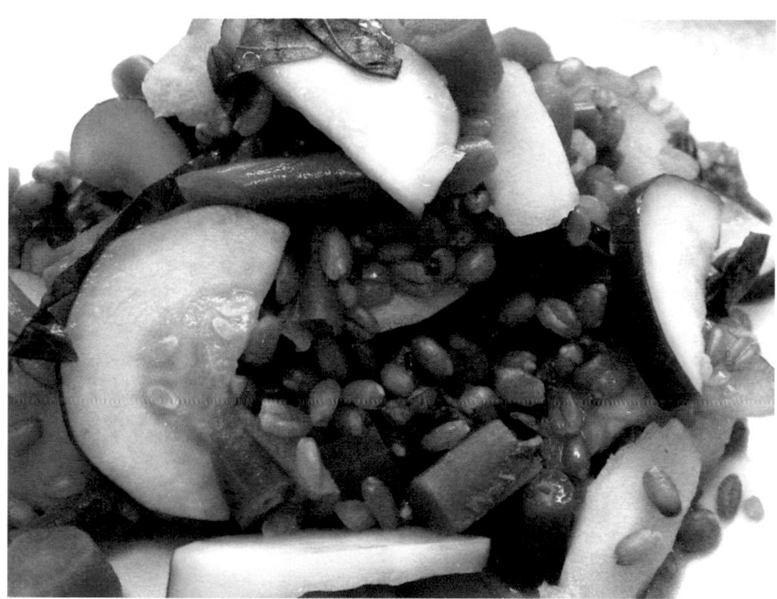

***Notes*** • *The chicken stock evaporates as you cook the vegetables, so it's important to keep a little extra on hand. If the stock is flavorful enough, you can add water instead.* • *The chicken cutlet can be prepared up to one day in advance. Cover and refrigerate.* • *It is important to use a sharp chef's knife when slicing the basil, or it gets crushed and quickly turns black.* • *Barley takes 15–20 minutes to cook. You can substitute wheat berries, which take 30–40 minutes and have a slightly chewy consistency.* • *The garlic used in the oil should be discarded. It imparts a toasted garlic flavor without actually leaving garlic in the food.* • *Make sure you cook the vegetables one at a time, as their cooking time varies.* • *After cooking the vegetables, keep the stock to add flavor to a soup of your choice.*

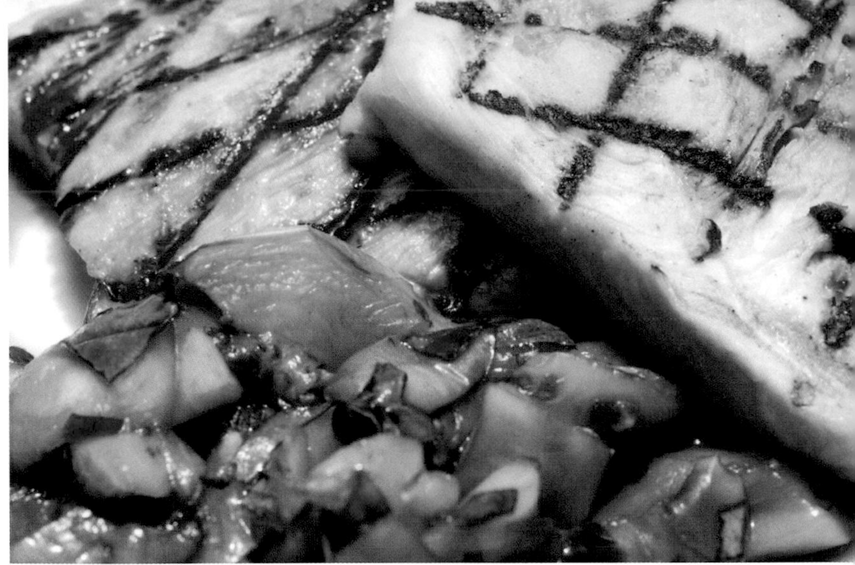

# Grilled Turkey Breast with Japanese Eggplant

***Serves 4***
***Nutritional information per serving***
Calories 366
Protein 59g
Carbohydrates 22g
Fat 7g

### Ingredients for the grilled turkey breast

4 slices turkey breast (about 8 oz each)
2 Tbsp miso paste
2 Tbsp honey
2 Tbsp fresh sage (washed, stems removed, chopped fine)

### Ingredients for the Japanese eggplant

1 lb Japanese eggplant (ends trimmed, cut in half lengthwise and then on the bias in ½-inch pieces)
1 Tbsp olive oil
1 Tbsp soy sauce
2 Tbsp plum sauce
2 Tbsp fresh basil (washed, stems removed, sliced thin)

### Directions for the turkey breast

1. Mix the honey, miso, and fine-chopped sage.
2. Add the turkey breast and marinate from 15 minutes to several hours.

### Directions for the Japanese eggplant

1. Heat a sauté pan over medium heat. Add olive oil and eggplant, and sear until golden brown, stirring often to avoid burning.
2. When golden brown, add soy sauce, plum sauce, and basil. Cover and cook slowly another 5 minutes. Keep warm.
3. Serve immediately with the turkey breast.

### To serve

1. Heat the grill pan to medium heat. Brush the pan with a grill brush and rub with a lightly oiled rag. The pan should smoke, but not flare up.
2. Drain and pat the turkey dry.
3. Place on the grill for 1 minute.
4. With a pair of tongs, lift the turkey and turn a few degrees off its original position to create diamond-shaped grill marks.
5. Repeat on the other side.

**Notes** • *I like the turkey breast cooked so that a light pink color can be seen when slicing it. Otherwise, the meat will be dry and chalky.* • *After cooking, let the turkey rest about 5 minutes so the juices redistribute throughout the breast. During cooking, the juices concentrate toward the middle of the meat.*

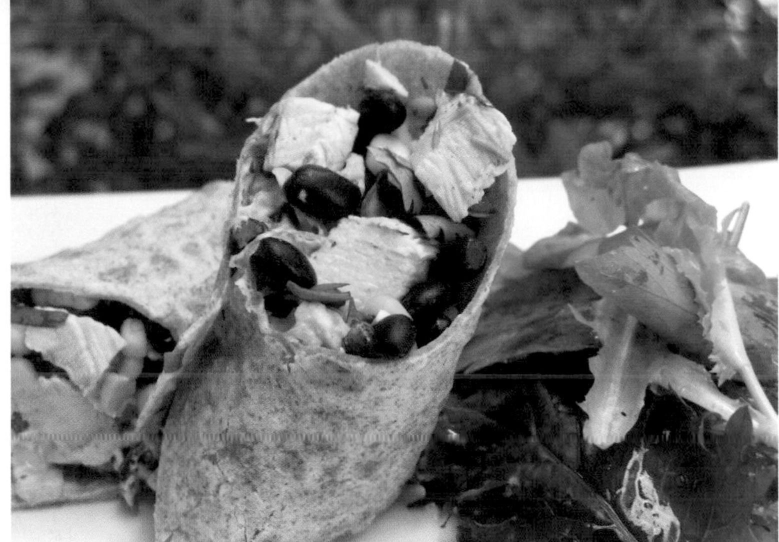

# Chicken South-of-the-Border Style

***Serves 4***
***Nutritional information per serving***
Calories 301
Protein 30g
Carbohydrates 34g
Fat 5g

## Ingredients

4 8-in whole-wheat tortillas
12 oz chicken breast (boneless and skinless)
1 tsp cumin
¼ cup cilantro leaves (washed, stems removed and chopped coarse)
¼ tsp lime zest (shaved with a microplane)
3 Tbsp nonfat sour cream
1 ear corn (kernels removed and simmered in chicken stock for 5 minutes, then drained)
1 cup canned black beans (drained)

## Directions

1. Combine the lime zest and the sour cream. Add the cumin, the chicken, and half the cilantro. Marinate for 20 minutes to 3 hours.
2. Preheat the grill. Brush it and then wipe the grill with a lightly oiled rag. If a flame flares up, there's too much oil on the rag.
3. Drain the excess marinade and pat the chicken breast dry.
4. Place the chicken on the grill and flip when golden brown. Lower the temperature if the grill marks are too dark and the chicken is still underdone.
5. Remove the chicken and let it cool slightly. Place on a cutting board and dice into ½-inch cubes. Reserve in a small bowl.

## To serve

1. Preheat a nonstick sauté pan on low heat.
2. Place the tortilla flat in the pan.
3. Dip a pastry brush in about 1 Tbsp water and brush over the tortilla.
4. When the bottom of the tortilla begins to turn golden brown, flip it over and place a quarter of the chicken, a pinch of cilantro, some sour cream, corn, and black beans on the tortilla.
5. Place the tortilla on a cutting board. Fold one inch of the right edge of the tortilla over toward the middle, then the left edge.
6. Starting at the unfolded edge, roll the tortilla into a burrito.
7. Serve immediately.

***Notes*** • *You can add more cilantro if you like more flavor.* • *When grilling the chicken, you can grill both sides quickly and finish cooking in the oven.*

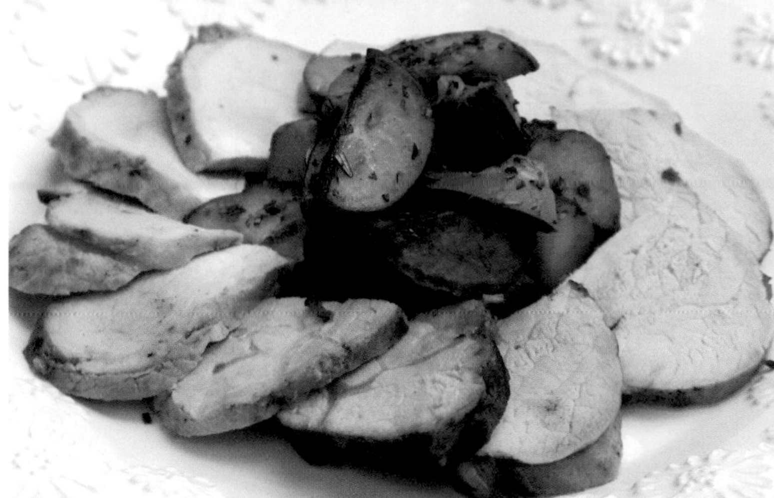

# Pork Loin with Fingerling Potatoes and Zucchini

*Serves 4*
***Nutritional information per serving***
Calories 493
Protein 41g
Carbohydrates 44g
Fat 17g

### Ingredients for the pork

1½ lbs lean pork loin (trim excess fat)
1 Tbsp canola oil

### Ingredients for the brine

1 qt water or chicken stock
1½ cups salt
6 whole cloves
6 bay leaves
10 juniper berries
¼ tsp cardamom

### Ingredients for the potatoes and zucchini

2 lbs fingerling potatoes (washed, dried, and cut into 1½-inch long sections, then on the bias, and dried prior to cooking)
1 small zucchini (about 1½ inches diameter, cut in half lengthwise, then sliced ⅛-inch thick)
2 Tbsp fresh thyme (stems removed, chopped fine)
2 Tbsp olive oil
1 Tbsp fresh rosemary (stems removed, chopped fine)
Salt

### Directions for the brine

1. Bring the water or chicken stock to a simmer with the salt, cloves, bay leaves, juniper berries, and cardamom.
2. Cook for 15 minutes and allow to cool.
3. When room temperature, place the pork in the brine and let sit for 1 to 12 hours (or overnight) in the refrigerator.

### Directions for the pork

1. Preheat the oven to 375°F.
2. Remove the pork from the brine.
3. Remove all aromatic garnish, and dry pork with paper towels.
4. Place a roasting pan on the top of the stove over medium-high heat. Add the canola oil, and when the oil begins to smoke, add the pork.
5. Place in the oven and bake until evenly browned.
6. Cook until the temperature reaches 140°F on a meat thermometer in the thickest part of the meat. It will take about 20–35 minutes.
7. Let rest for 10 minutes.

### Directions for the potatoes and zucchini

1. Place the oil in a pan over low to medium heat. Add the dried potatoes and cook for 10 minutes, stirring often or until golden brown.
2. Add the zucchini, rosemary, thyme, and salt. Cook another 5 minutes until the herbs are mixed thoroughly and the zucchini is al dente.

***Notes*** • *It is always important to let roasted meat rest for about a third of the time it takes to cook, so that the juices that concentrated toward the middle can redistribute to the edges. If the meat is cut immediately, the juices run out and the meat becomes dry.* • *Do not cook the pork over high heat, as the meat will dry out and toughen.*

*Serves 2*
***Nutritional information per serving***
Calories 477
Protein 34g
Carbohydrates 57g
Fat 12g

### Ingredients

8 oz pork tenderloin (or lean pork loin with fat removed, cut into 1½-inch strips)
½ cup broccoli (cut into florets about the size of a cherry)
2 cups Japanese eggplant (cut in half lengthwise and sliced thin crosswise)
1 cup mushrooms (washed, drained, ¼ inch removed from the base of the stem, then cut in quarters)
1 cup asparagus (1-inch pieces; discard the bottom 3 inches of stem unless peeled)
1 cup snow peas (cleaned, ends removed and cut on the bias into 3 pieces)
1 cup carrots (cut in half lengthwise, then into slices on the bias)
3 Tbsp fresh basil (washed, dried, and sliced thin with a sharp knife)
3 Tbsp fresh ginger (peeled and sliced thin)
2 Tbsp oyster sauce
2 tsp fish sauce
2 tsp soy sauce
4 lime leaves
1 Tbsp oil
1 cup chicken stock
3 oz Chinese rice vermicelli (soaked in cold water 15 minutes)

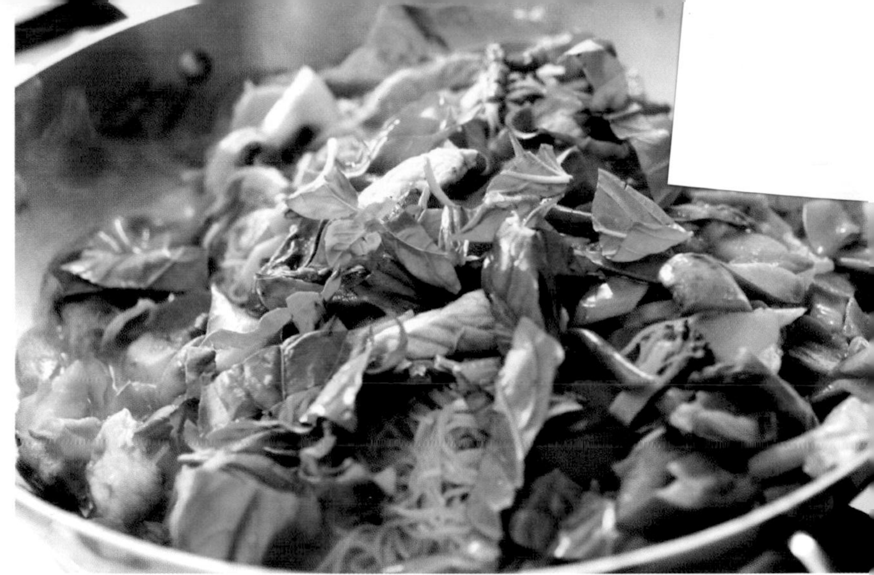

# Asian Pork Stir-Fry

### Directions

1. Cut all vegetables into bite-sized pieces.
2. Place the oil in a large shallow pan with a tight-fitting lid.
3. Over medium to high heat, add the ginger and carrots. Cook until slightly golden brown.
4. Add the broccoli, Japanese eggplant, mushrooms, asparagus, snow peas, lime leaves, and half of the chicken stock.
5. Cover with a lid and cook 4-6 minutes.
6. When vegetables are al dente, add the other half of the chicken stock. Place the soaked vermicelli on top. Cover and cook on high another 3 minutes.
7. When the pasta becomes tender and soft but still has texture, add the pork, oyster sauce, soy sauce, and fish sauce. Lower the temperature. Add the basil and mix the vermicelli into the vegetables.
8. If the mixture seems dry, add another ½ cup water or chicken stock.
9. The pork is cooked when the meat has no traces of red.
10. Serve on a plate by removing the vermicelli with tongs and place on a plate with the vegetables on top.

**Notes** • *Lime leaves or kaffir leaves are found in Asian markets. They can be kept in the freezer for months. Just two or three leaves are sufficient to add perfume to a dish.* • *I like the ginger in slices, as I like to taste that bite of ginger flavor.* • *The pork is added at the end of the recipe so it remains moist.* • *You can substitute boneless, skinless chicken breast, cut the same way.* • *The soy sauce, oyster sauce, and fish sauce are added at the end because they caramelize and burn easily.*

# Spaghetti with White Clam Sauce

***Serves 4***
***Nutritional information per serving***
Calories 603
Protein 43g
Carbohydrates 83g
Fat 12g

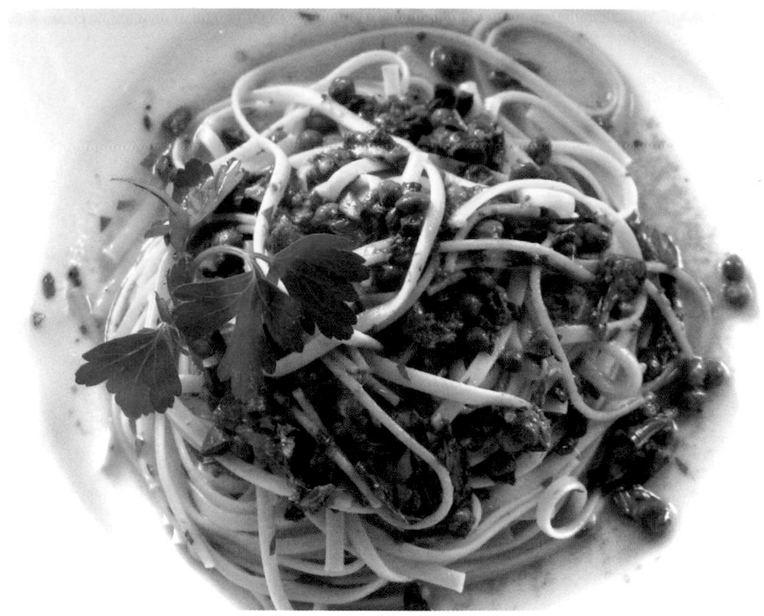

## Ingredients

- 1 lb whole-wheat spaghetti
- 2 cans canned clams (4-oz can)
- 1 bottle clam juice (about 8 fl oz)
- ½ cup fresh parsley (washed, stems removed, chopped coarse and dried)
- 2 Tbsp extra-virgin olive oil
- 1 tsp salt
- 1 tsp ginger (peeled and grated fine with a microplane)
- ¼ tsp lemon zest (washed and grated fine with a microplane)

## Directions

1. Bring a pot of salted water to a boil. Add the pasta and cook 7–8 minutes. Drain.
2. In a pan over medium heat, add the olive oil and ginger. Cook for 2 minutes.
3. Add the clams, ½ of the clam juice, the parsley, and the lemon zest. Bring to a simmer.
4. Add the pasta and mix with a pair of tongs.
5. Add salt to taste.
6. Add the rest of the clam juice, if necessary.
7. Serve in a soup bowl by twisting the pasta with a pair of tongs or a chef's fork.
8. Pour the clams and juice from the bottom of the bowl over the pasta.

***Notes*** • *Whole-wheat pasta has a more al dente texture than regular pasta. Whole wheat is a healthier alternative, as it doesn't assimilate in the body as quickly, thus keeping you satisfied longer. It can be cooked 2–3 minutes longer than regular pasta.* • *I like to drain the pasta after cooking without cooling it in cold water.* • *I use imported dry pasta. The quality is consistent and stays al dente if cooked 7–8 minutes.*

# Crusted Cod with Beans and Carrots

***Serves 4***
***Nutritional information per serving***
Calories 228
Protein 17g
Carbohydrates 35g
Fat 4g

## Ingredients

- 4 slices of cod filet, about 7 oz each (ask your fishmonger to remove skin and bones)
- 1 Tbsp fresh thyme (wash, dry, remove leaves from sprigs and chop fine)
- 1 cup flour
- 1 egg (beat in a bowl with fork, adding a pinch of salt; do not whip air into it)
- ½ package kataifi (shredded filo dough; cut in 2-inch sections, mix gently in a bowl, and spread evenly, about 4 oz per plate)
- 2 Tbsp olive oil
- 1 pint chicken stock (16 fl oz)
- 1 Tbsp soy sauce
- 2 lime leaves
- 3 Tbsp capers
- 2 tsp ginger
- ¼ lb peeled baby carrots or young market carrots (trim the ends and cut into ¼-inch thick pieces)
- 1 dozen Little Neck clams (rinse in cold water)
- ¼ cup fresh parsley (washed, dried and chopped fine)
- 1 lb fava beans (fresh or frozen)
- 1 lb cannellini beans
- Salt to taste

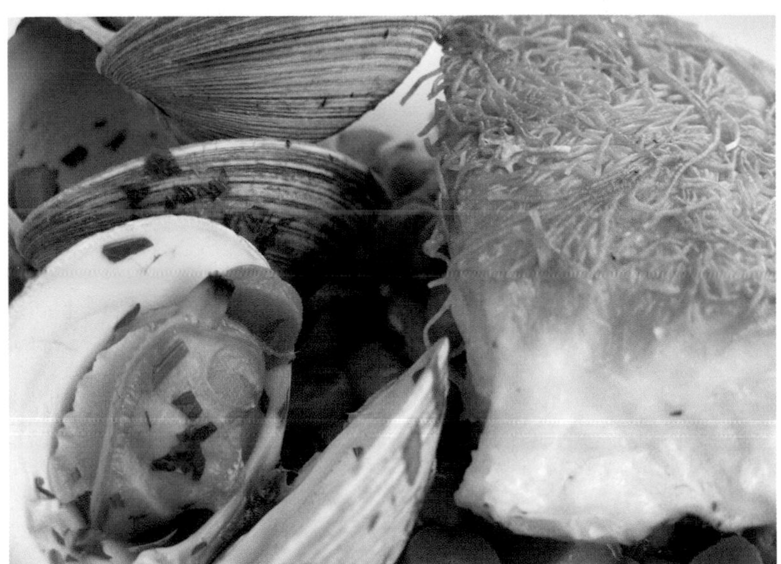

## Directions

1. Season both sides of the codfish with salt and thyme.
2. Dip one side of the codfish steak in the flour and shake off the excess.
3. Dip the same side in the egg wash and drain the excess.
4. Dip the same side in the kataifi (only on one side).
5. Place a medium-sized nonstick pan on the stove, medium heat.
6. Add the olive oil and the 4 portions of codfish (kataifi side down).
7. Cook about 7–10 minutes on low heat.
8. Flip and cook another 3 minutes.
9. Remove and drain off excess fat on paper towels; keep warm.
10. Wipe the pan with paper towels.
11. Add the chicken stock and bring to a boil.
12. Add the soy sauce, lime leaves, capers, ginger, carrots, and clams. Cover with a tight lid and simmer for 5 minutes, until clams open up.
13. Add the parsley, fava, and cannellini beans and adjust seasonings.
14. Remove lime leaves.
15. Place the broth with the beans, clams, and carrots in a soup bowl, and place the crisp codfish on top.

***Notes*** • *Only dip one side of the cod in the kataifi so it cooks to a beautiful golden brown color and can be used as the presentation side.* • *The goal in sautéing the codfish on low heat is to sear the crust to a golden color just until the flesh coagulates. If cooked properly, it will remain flaky and moist.* • *You can replace the baby fava beans with frozen soybeans. Fava beans are usually available in the spring and summer. Frozen fava beans can be used in winter.*

# Asian-Style Shrimp with Jasmine Rice

*Serves 4*
***Nutritional information per serving***
Calories 447
Protein 36g
Carbohydrates 33g
Fat 18g

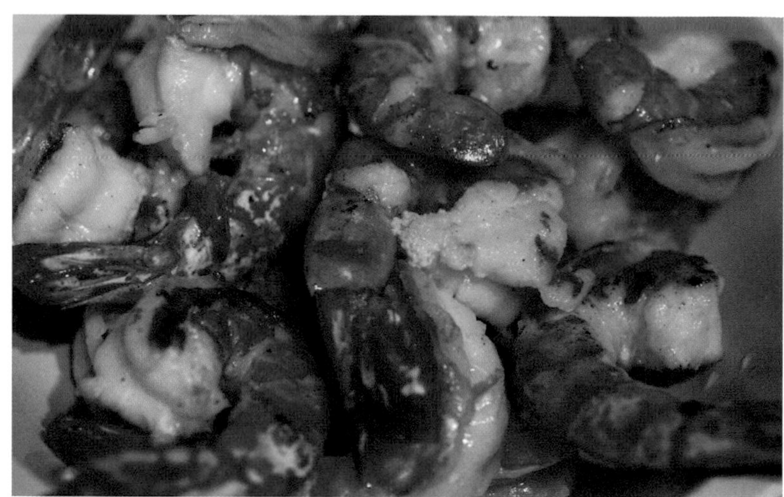

### Ingredients for the Asian-style shrimp

2 Tbsp butter
1 lb shrimp (size 16–20/lb) (peeled, deveined, and rinsed)
2 Tbsp fresh cilantro (washed, dried, stems removed, chopped coarse)
2 Tbsp fresh basil (washed, dried, stems removed, chopped coarse)
1 bottle clam juice (about 8 fl oz)
2 tsp fish sauce (nam pla) (mixed in a small bowl with the cornstarch)
¼ tsp cornstarch
1 tsp brown sugar
¼ tsp salt
¼ tsp sesame oil

### Ingredients for the jasmine rice

1½ cup jasmine rice (rinse for 1 minute under cold water)
1¾ cup chicken stock
1 tsp ground coriander
1 tsp salt

### Directions for the jasmine rice

1. Place the ground coriander in a sauté pan over medium heat. As soon as the coriander fragrance dissipates, add the chicken stock. Remove from heat.
2. Pour the coriander and stock into a saucepan.
3. Add the rice and salt. Bring to a simmer.
4. Cover and cook about 20 minutes on a very low simmer.
5. Stir gently when cooked and keep covered until needed.

### Directions for the shrimp

1. Place a sauté pan over medium heat. Add the butter and shrimp.
2. Cook about 3 minutes on each side until shrimp turns opaque.
3. Remove the shrimp. Cover and reserve.
4. Add the clam juice, fish sauce, cornstarch, sugar, and salt.
5. Bring to a boil and stir with a whisk to keep it from sticking to the sides of the pan.
6. When the sauce has reduced by half, return the shrimp to the pan.
7. Add the cilantro, basil, and sesame oil. Serve immediately, with the jasmine rice on the side.

***Notes*** • *It's safe to cook the rice before the shrimp, as it takes about 25 minutes to cook and rest.* • *Jasmine rice is very delicate. Don't stir it too much once it's cooked, or it will break apart.* • *Stirring the fish sauce into the cornstarch allows the sauce to thicken without lumps.* • *Always devein shrimp. The size of the vein can vary; it may be thick in one shrimp and practically nonexistent in another.*

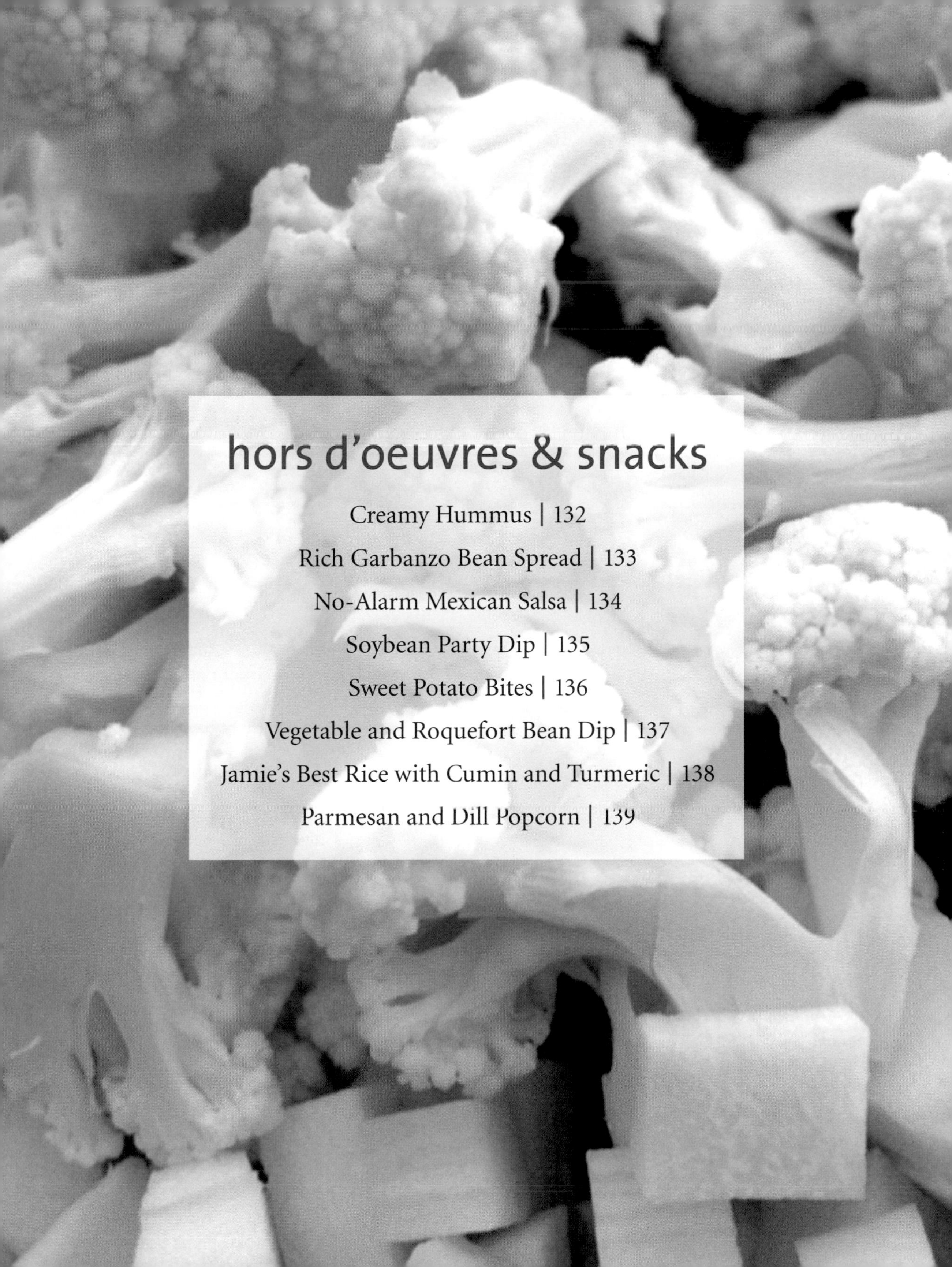

# hors d'oeuvres & snacks


Creamy Hummus | 132

Rich Garbanzo Bean Spread | 133

No-Alarm Mexican Salsa | 134

Soybean Party Dip | 135

Sweet Potato Bites | 136

Vegetable and Roquefort Bean Dip | 137

Jamie's Best Rice with Cumin and Turmeric | 138

Parmesan and Dill Popcorn | 139

# Creamy Hummus

***Serves 24***
***Nutritional information per serving***
Calories 38
Protein 1g
Carbohydrates 5g
Fat 1g

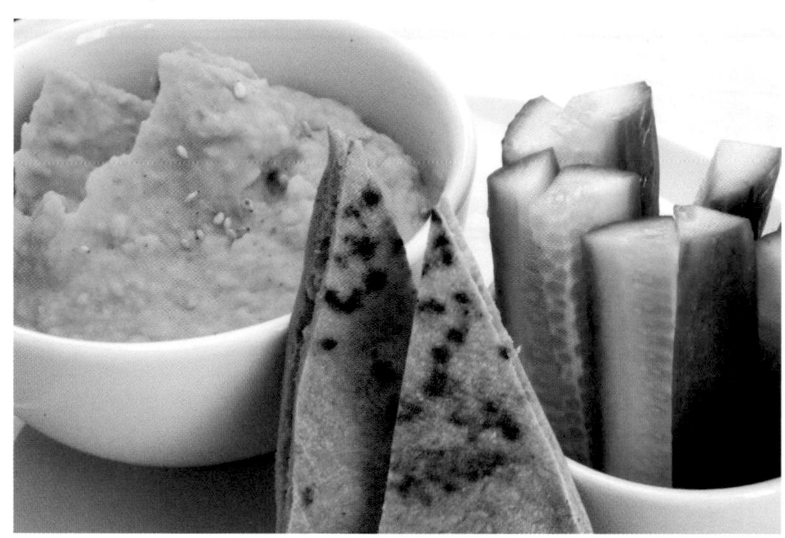

## Ingredients

- 1 can (19 oz) canned chickpeas (drained and washed twice)
- 1 cup chicken stock
- 2 Tbsp olive oil
- ¼ tsp sesame oil
- ½ tsp salt

## Directions

1. Place the chickpeas in a food processor and add the chicken stock, olive oil, sesame oil, and salt.
2. Process until smooth.
3. Add chicken stock as needed.
4. Serve cold with toast points, oven-toasted corn chips, or small wedges of flatbread.

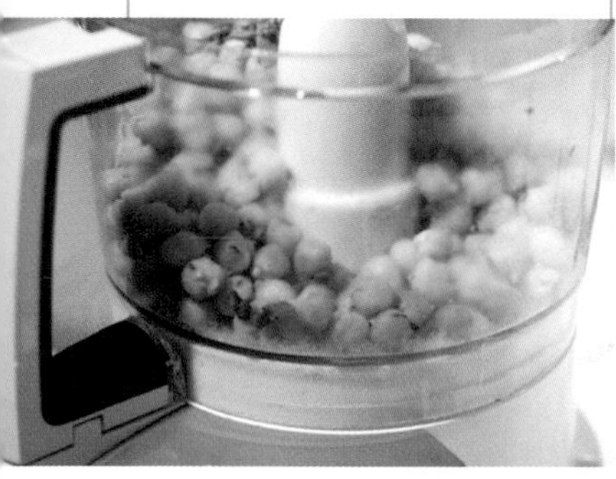

***Notes*** • *I like to rinse the beans twice to remove excess starch.* • *Depending on how you like the consistency, you can use more or less chicken stock.*

***Serves 24***
***Nutritional information per serving***
Calories 49
Protein 3g
Carbohydrates 6g
Fat 2g

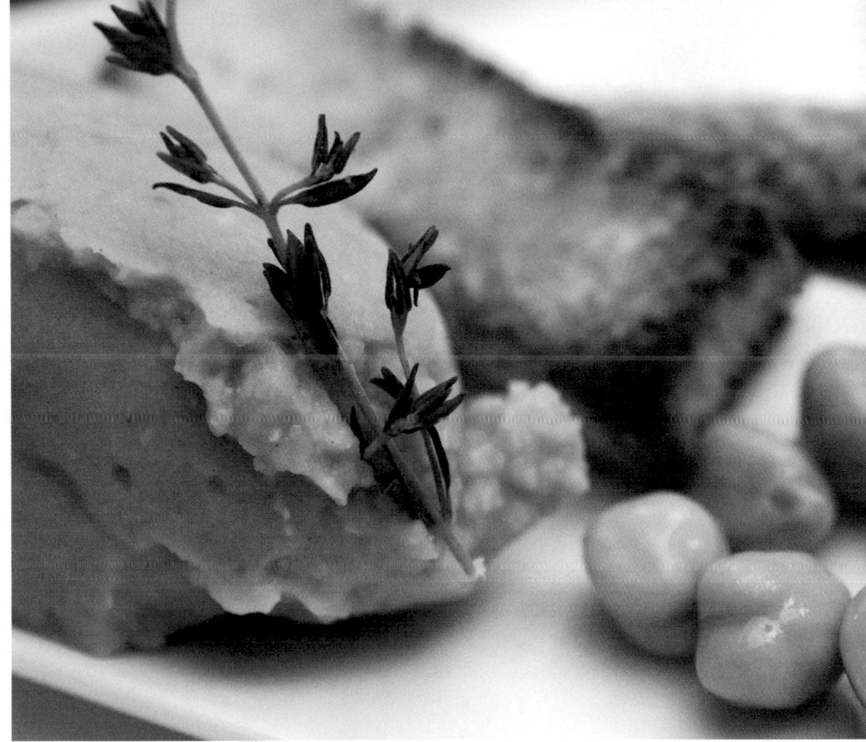

# Rich Garbanzo Bean Spread

## Ingredients

1¼ cups garbanzo beans (soaked in water for a couple of hours or overnight in the refrigerator)
3 qt chicken stock
2 oz (4 slices) prosciutto
1 bay leaf
2 branches fresh thyme
2 Tbsp sesame seeds, toasted golden brown
Salt to taste

## Directions

1. Drain the water from the beans and place them with 2½ qt of the chicken stock in a medium pot.
2. Add the slices of prosciutto, the bay leaf, and the thyme. Place a cover over ¾ of the pot and simmer about 2 hours.
3. If the stock reduces to a level below the beans, add more stock to cover.
4. When the beans are soft, drain them. Remove the bay leaves, thyme, and prosciutto. Cool and place in a food processor with the sesame seeds, and process until smooth.
5. Add salt and chicken stock as needed for the desired consistency.
6. Serve cold with toast points, oven-toasted corn chips, or small wedges of flatbread.

**Notes** • *You can simplify the procedure by using an 8 oz can of chickpeas. If you do, rinse twice under cold water and process in a food processor until smooth. It will save 2 hours, but you sacrifice some flavor. If you add salt while cooking the beans, the cooking time will be lengthened by several hours, as the outside skin of the chickpeas will not soften.* • *For added flavor, the prosciutto can be processed with the beans; it will not be as smooth, though.* • *The traditional hummus recipe calls for tahini, which is a paste of roasted sesame seeds. Since it is not always available, we've substituted freshly toasted sesame seeds.*

# No-Alarm Mexican Salsa

*Serves 20*
***Nutritional information per serving***
Calories 30
Protein 1g
Carbohydrates 3g
Fat 2g

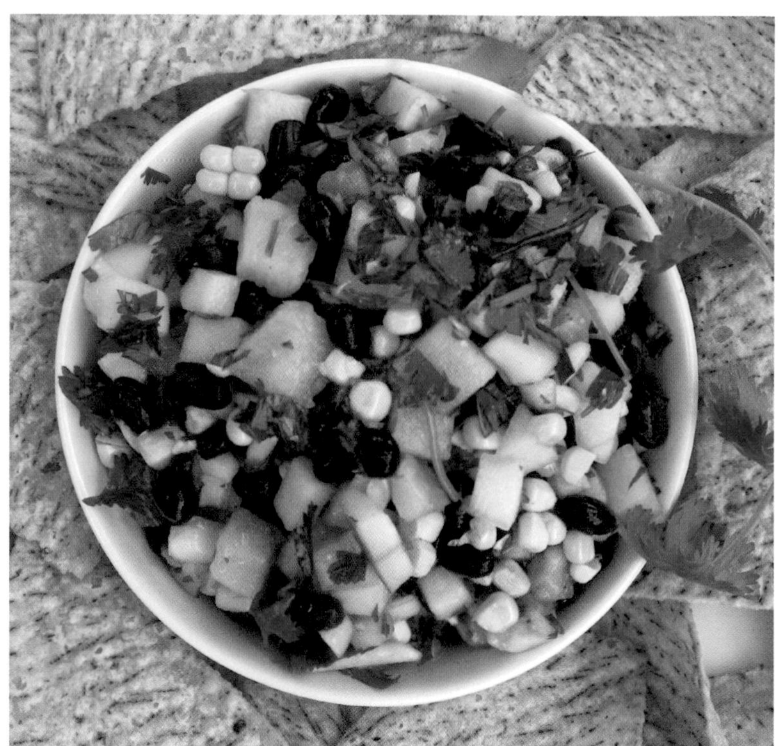

## Ingredients

- ½ cup corn kernels (fresh or canned)
- ½ cup cucumber (washed, cut in half, seeds removed, and diced into ¼-inch cubes)
- ½ cup banana (peeled and diced into ¼-inch cubes)
- ½ cup pineapple (fresh, peeled, cut in half lengthwise, then in quarters, core removed, and diced into ¼-inch cubes)
- ½ cup canned black beans (rinsed and drained)
- 1 avocado, sliced and diced
- Optional: ½ cup honeydew (skin and seeds removed, then diced into ¼-inch cubes)
- ¼ tsp fresh ginger, grated
- ½ tsp ground cumin (best if whole cumin is roasted in a pan and ground when needed)
- 2 Tbsp fresh parsley (washed, stems removed, dried and chopped fine)
- 2 Tbsp fresh cilantro (washed, stems removed, dried and chopped coarse)
- 2 Tbsp extra-virgin olive oil
- ¼ cup pineapple juice
- 1 tsp salt, or more to taste

## Directions

1. Place the corn, cucumber, banana, pineapple, black beans, honeydew, ginger, cumin, parsley, cilantro, olive oil, and pineapple juice in a bowl.
2. Mix thoroughly and season with salt.
3. Add the avocado last, as it can easily become mashed.
4. Serve immediately before the bright green color of the herbs fades.

***Notes*** • *If you don't mind the herbs turning a darker green, you can let it sit for half an hour, allowing the flavors to blend.* • *Fresh corn tastes especially good during the summer season, when it is sweet.* • *You can simplify the recipe by omitting the aloe vera, avocado, and honeydew.* • *To keep the avocado green, pour some of the pineapple juice over it.* • *This recipe is best served cold. If you don't serve immediately, keep refrigerated, or the chlorophyll will blacken.* • *This salsa is delicious with fish.*

# Soybean Party Dip

***Serves 20***
***Nutritional information per serving***
Calories 30
Protein 2g
Carbohydrates 2g
Fat 1g

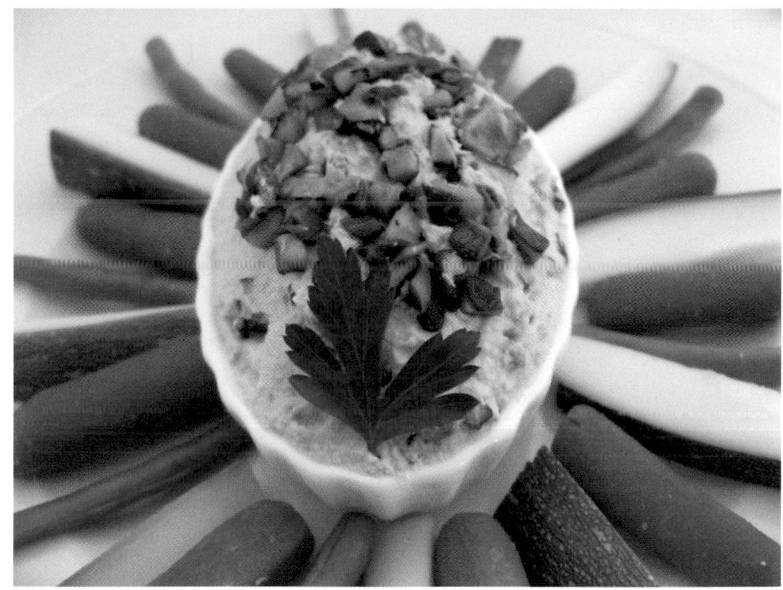

## Ingredients

1 lb pressed firm tofu (preferably House Premium Tofu)
2 Tbsp toasted sesame seeds
1 Tbsp white miso paste
1 Tbsp honey
2 tsp light soy sauce
1 tsp fresh ginger (peeled and grated fine with a microplane)
1 cup (3 oz) shitake mushrooms (stems removed, washed, diced in ⅓-inch cubes)
2 tsp olive oil
Salt to taste

Zucchini, cauliflower, and snow peas, or dipping vegetables of your choice

## Directions

1. Heat a sauté pan over medium heat with 2 tsp olive oil. Add the mushrooms and sauté until all the juice has evaporated. Season with salt to taste. Let cool.
2. Place the tofu, sesame seeds, miso paste, honey, soy sauce, and ginger in a blender. Blend until smooth. Pour into a serving dish.
3. Add the shitake mushrooms.
4. Sprinkle with fresh or dried herbs of your choice.

***Notes*** • *Perhaps the name of this dip does not suggest that it is delicious, but it is. The shitake mushrooms on the top add a wonderful texture.* • *We like to serve it with vegetables, although it could be served with crackers as well.*

# Sweet Potato Bites

*Serves 8*
*Nutritional information per serving*
Calories 66
Protein 1g
Carbohydrates 15g
Fat 0.5g

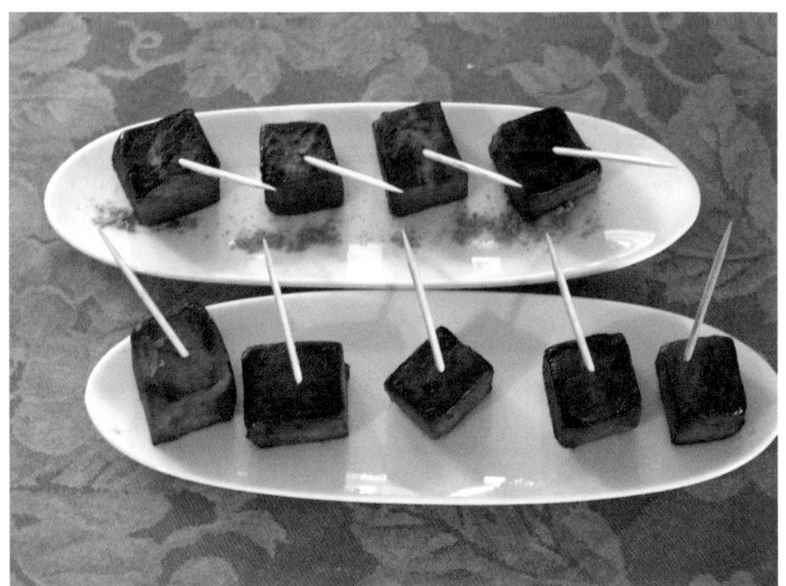

## Ingredients

2 large sweet potatoes (peeled, rinsed, and diced into 1-inch cubes)
1 Tbsp low-sodium soy sauce
1 Tbsp honey
5 sprigs thyme (washed, stems removed, and chopped fine)
Nonstick spray (about ½ tsp)

## Directions

1. In a bowl, mix the soy sauce, thyme, and honey.
2. Add the cubed potatoes and let stand for 1 minute.
3. Heat a nonstick pan over medium heat. Spray with nonstick spray.
4. Drain the potatoes, dry slightly with a paper towel, and place in the pan in a single layer. Brown all sides and, if not tender, finish in a 350°F oven for about 10 minutes.

## To serve

You can serve the potatoes in a flat ceramic dish with toothpicks.

**Notes** • *If the potatoes are getting too brown in the pan, lower the heat and finish in the oven at 350°F.* • *To speed up the cooking process, cover with a lid so the heat is dispersed more evenly throughout the pan.* • *If you like your snack a touch sweeter, you can pour extra honey or maple syrup over the cooked potatoes.*

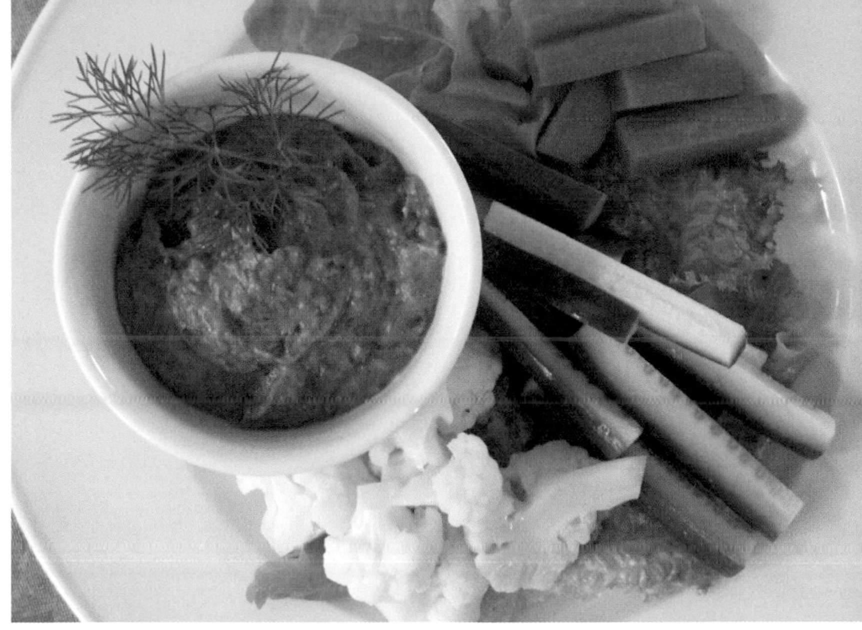

# Vegetable and Roquefort Bean Dip

***Serves 17***
***Nutritional information per serving***
Calories 33
Protein 2g
Carbohydrates 6g
Fat 0.2g

### Ingredients for the bean dip

1 can (14 oz) red beans
1 Tbsp Roquefort cheese (or gorgonzola)
10 sprigs flat-leaf parsley (washed, stems removed, chopped fine and dried)
1 Tbsp chicken stock

### Ingredients for the vegetables

½ lb (2 cups) seedless cucumber or Persian cucumber (washed and cut the size of French fries)
½ lb (1½ cups) young market carrots (or substitute "baby carrots") (washed, peeled, and both ends removed)

### Directions for the bean dip

1. Drain the beans and place in a blender. Add the chicken stock and half the cheese. Blend to the desired consistency.
2. Pour into a bowl, add the parsley, and mix thoroughly with a wooden spoon or rubber spatula. Sprinkle with the remainder of the cheese. Stir to combine.
3. Serve in a ramekin or small serving bowl.
4. The vegetables should be chilled and kept covered until the last minute so they stay fresh.

***Notes*** • *In the spring or fall, if you find young carrots with the greens on, keep about two inches of the greens and remove just the wilted leaves. It will give the carrots more flavor.*

# Jamie's Best Rice with Cumin and Turmeric

***Serves 4***
***Nutritional information per serving***
Calories 127
Protein 4g
Carbohydrates 19g
Fat 4g

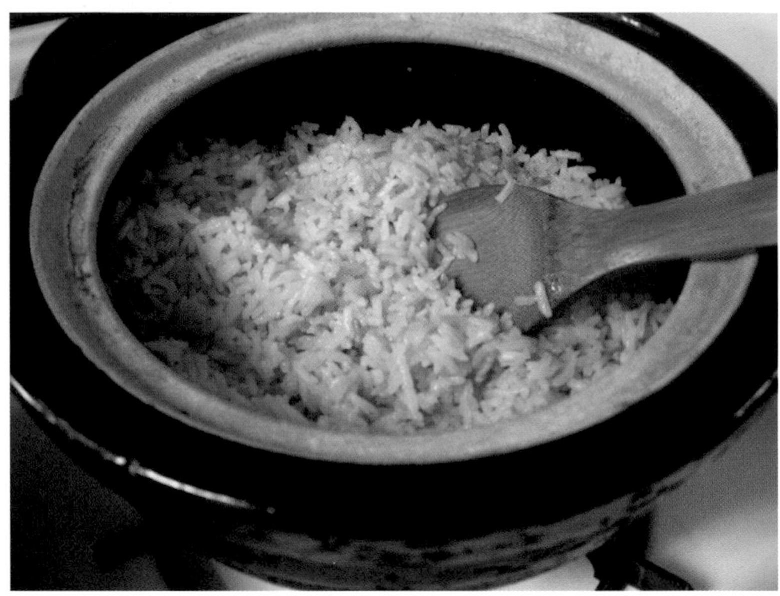

## Ingredients

1 cup jasmine rice
1 can (14 oz) chicken broth
1 cup water
1 Tbsp salad oil
¼ tsp salt
¼ tsp ground cumin
¼ tsp turmeric

## Directions

1. Spray a rice cooker with nonstick spray and add the salad oil, rice, water, and chicken broth.
2. Add the seasonings and stir the ingredients.
3. Start the rice cooker 30–45 minutes before you plan on serving.
4. Stir once, about 10 minutes into the cooking process.
5. Fluff immediately after the rice cooker turns off.
6. Keep covered until ready to serve.

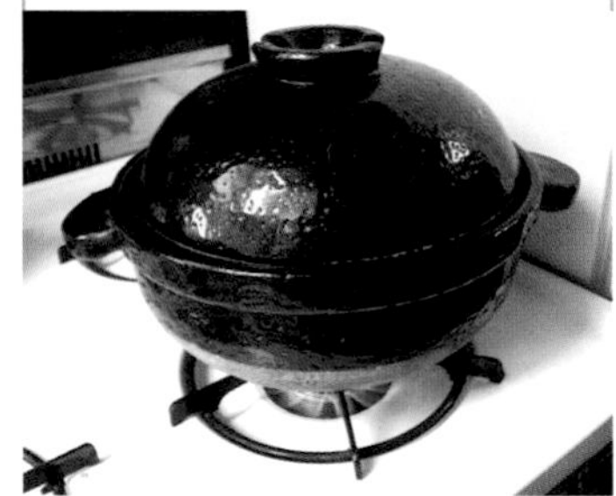

**Notes** • *Use a rice cooker. If you don't have one, they're relatively inexpensive.* • *This rice dish is a beautiful golden color and goes great with almost everything, especially fish.* • *I use jasmine rice because it isn't sticky, and my preferred ratio of liquid to rice is 3:2.*

# Parmesan and Dill Popcorn

*Serves 10*
***Nutritional information per serving***
Calories 32
Protein 1g
Carbohydrates 4g
Fat 2g

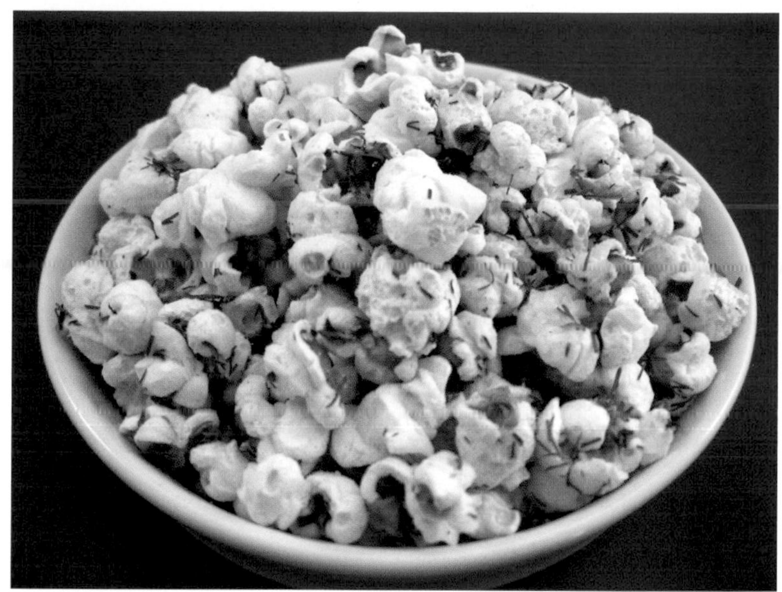

## Ingredients

1 cup popping-corn kernels
1 Tbsp olive oil
1 Tbsp grated Parmesan cheese
2 Tbsp fresh dill (washed, stems removed, and chopped fine)

## Directions

1. Heat a pan that is large enough to hold the corn in a single layer over medium heat.
2. Add the oil and the corn and stir until the corn starts to pop (about 3–5 minutes).
3. Cover the pan and lower the temperature.
4. Once the popcorn has stopped popping, remove from heat immediately.
5. Pour the corn into a bowl, then sprinkle with the grated Parmesan and fine-chopped dill.
6. Stir the cheese and herbs to mix evenly.
7. Serve promptly.

***Notes*** • *Make sure the pan is preheated before adding the oil and corn. Remove the corn that has not popped.* • *You can omit the dill or replace it with an herb of your choice.*

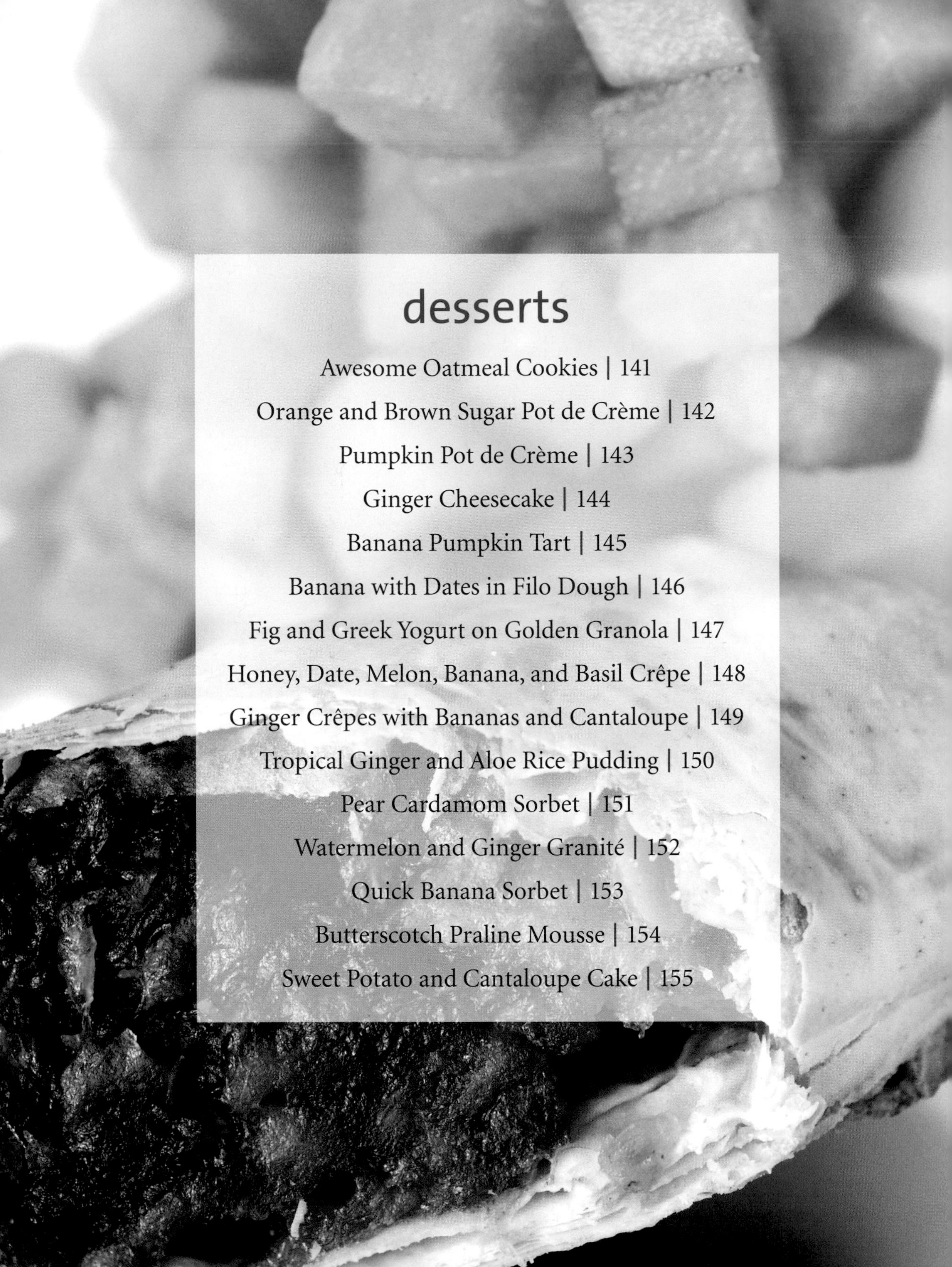

# desserts


Awesome Oatmeal Cookies | 141

Orange and Brown Sugar Pot de Crème | 142

Pumpkin Pot de Crème | 143

Ginger Cheesecake | 144

Banana Pumpkin Tart | 145

Banana with Dates in Filo Dough | 146

Fig and Greek Yogurt on Golden Granola | 147

Honey, Date, Melon, Banana, and Basil Crêpe | 148

Ginger Crêpes with Bananas and Cantaloupe | 149

Tropical Ginger and Aloe Rice Pudding | 150

Pear Cardamom Sorbet | 151

Watermelon and Ginger Granité | 152

Quick Banana Sorbet | 153

Butterscotch Praline Mousse | 154

Sweet Potato and Cantaloupe Cake | 155

# Awesome Oatmeal Cookies

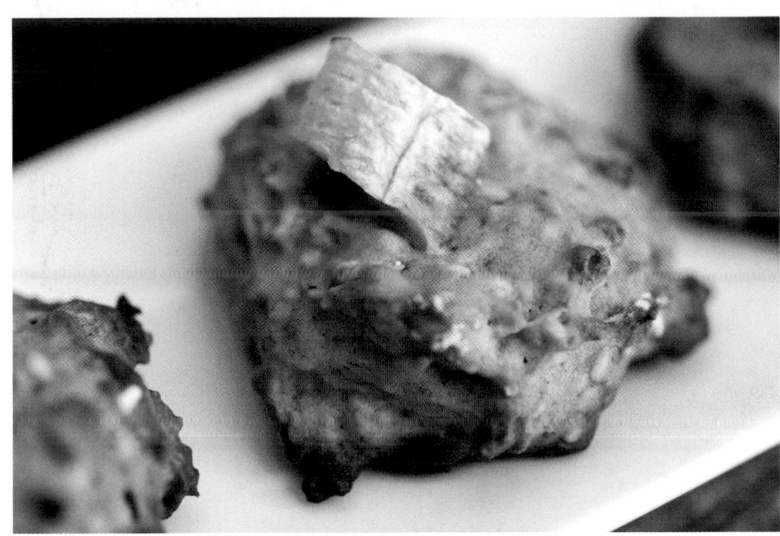

***Makes 40 cookies***
***Nutritional information per serving***
Calories per cookie 84
Protein 2g
Carbohydrates 12g
Fat 1g

### Ingredients

3 ripe bananas (blend until smooth)
½ cup brown sugar
2 whole eggs
¼ tsp salt
2 cups flour
1 tsp vanilla extract
½ tsp baking powder
1 cup instant rolled oats
¼ cup sesame seeds (toasted in a pan on the top of the stove until golden brown)
¼ banana cut in small pieces or 1 oz dark raisins (simmered in water for 10 minutes to rehydrate) for garnish on top of the cookies

### Directions

1. In a bowl, add the bananas, sugar, eggs, salt, vanilla, and sesame seeds.
2. In a separate bowl, mix the dry ingredients: flour, baking powder, and rolled oats.
3. Add the dry ingredients to the banana mix in 3 stages by folding dry into wet with a rubber spatula.
4. Spray nonstick coating on a cookie sheet.
5. Place 1 tsp cookie mix on the cookie sheet. Keep cookies about 2 inches apart.
6. Place a small dice of banana or some raisins on top of each cookie.
7. Cook in a preheated oven set at 350°F for 10–15 minutes or until the cookies turn a light golden color.
8. Remove from oven, let cool and enjoy.

***Notes*** • *These cookies aren't pretty, but they sure are delicious and good for* ***The Reflux Diet.***

# Orange and Brown Sugar Pot de Crème

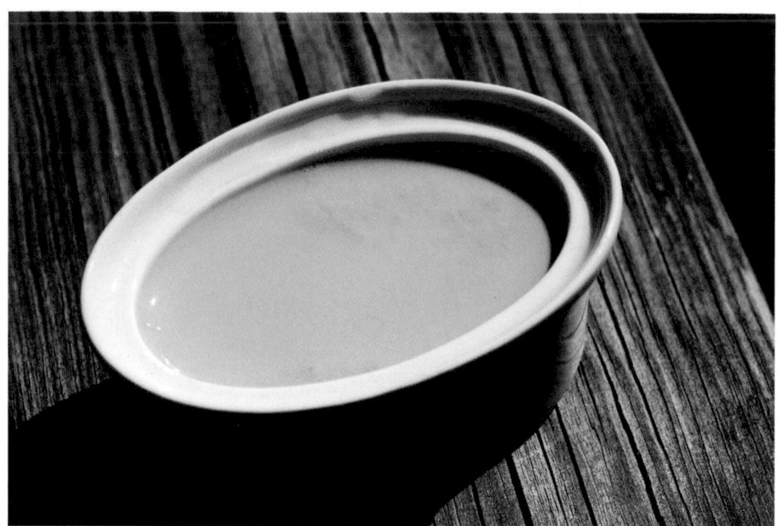

***Serves 5***
***Nutritional information per serving***
Calories 140
Protein 4g
Carbohydrates 25g
Fat 2g

## Ingredients

- 1 pint (8 fl oz) whole milk
- ½ cup brown sugar
- 2 eggs
- 1 tsp vanilla extract
- 1 tsp orange zest, washed and grated
- ¼ tsp salt

## Directions

1. Preheat oven to 325°F.
2. In a medium saucepan, bring the milk to a simmer with the orange zest, then remove from heat and infuse for about 10 minutes.
3. Using a fork, whisk the vanilla extract, brown sugar, salt, and eggs in a bowl.
4. Whisk in the milk and then strain through a fine strainer.
5. To remove excess foam, drag small squares of paper towel over the custard. Repeat the procedure until the custard is free of foam.
6. Pour the custard into 5 ramekins (3½ oz ramekins), up to ⅛ inch from the rim.
7. Place the ramekins in a gratin or casserole dish.
8. Fill the gratin dish with simmering water about halfway up the sides of the ramekins.
9. Place in the oven and bake until the custard is set, about 30–45 minutes.
10. When the custard is almost set, it will start to thicken. Remove from oven and cool to room temperature.
11. Store in refrigerator or serve immediately.

***Notes*** • *Straining the custard removes eggshells or unmixed egg white.* • *Using a fork to whisk the eggs will prevent too much foam from developing.* • *If you see the edges or center rising while baking the custard, remove immediately. It means that the custard has overcooked.*

*Serves 5*
***Nutritional information per serving***
Calories 175
Protein 4g
Carbohydrates 34g
Fat 3g

# Pumpkin Pot de Crème

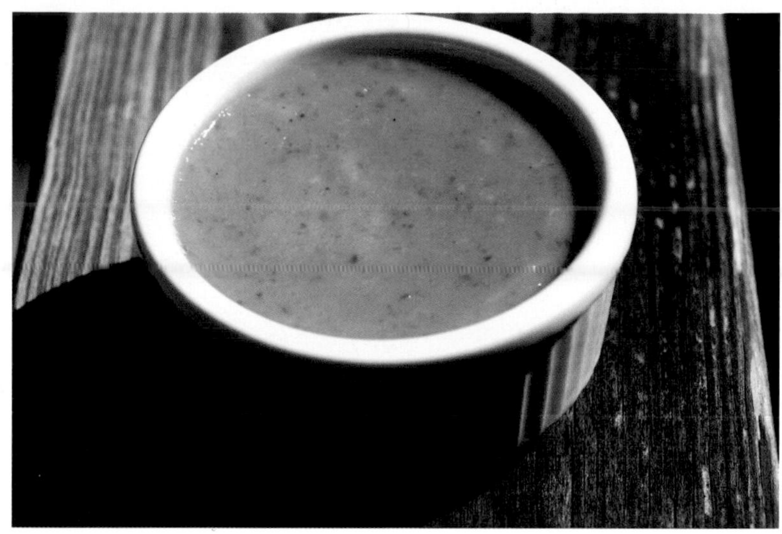

### Ingredients

1 cup (8 oz) pumpkin purée
1 cup whole milk
1 tsp fresh ginger (peeled and grated fine)
1⁄16 tsp ground cloves
⅛ tsp nutmeg
1¼ cups brown sugar
2 egg yolks
½ tsp vanilla extract
⅛ tsp salt
1 Tbsp pumpkin seeds, toasted

### Directions

1. Preheat oven to 325°F.
2. In a medium saucepan, bring the milk to a simmer with the ginger, cloves, and nutmeg.
3. Using a fork, whisk the egg yolks, sugar, salt, and vanilla in a bowl.
4. Add the pumpkin purée to the bowl.
5. Add the milk to the egg and pumpkin mix.
6. Pour the custard into ramekins (3 ½ oz ramekins) up to ⅛ inch from the rim.
7. Place the ramekins in a gratin or casserole dish.
8. Fill the gratin dish with simmering water about halfway up the sides of the ramekins.
9. Place in the oven and bake until the custard is set, about 30–45 minutes.
10. When the custard is almost set, it will start to thicken. Remove from oven and let cool to room temperature.
11. To serve, sprinkle with toasted pumpkin seeds.

***Notes*** • *This pot de crème is amazingly rich considering it is only 175 calories per serving.* • *The combination of pumpkin, ginger, and cloves makes it power-packed with flavor.*

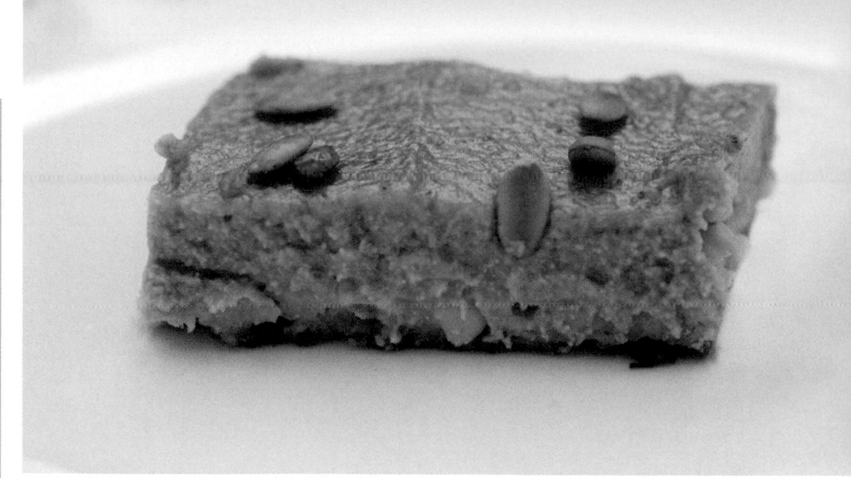

# Ginger Cheesecake

***Serves 8***
***Nutritional information per serving***
Calories 172
Protein 7g
Carbohydrates 22g
Fat 6g

### Ingredients for the filling
1 cup extra-firm tofu
1 cup (8 oz) pumpkin purée
½ cup cream cheese
1 tsp grated ginger
½ cup agave syrup or honey
¼ tsp salt

### Ingredients for the crust
½ cup polenta (instant polenta)
2½ cups milk
1 Tbsp sugar
1 tsp vanilla extract
¼ tsp salt
1 cup corn kernels
Nonstick spray

### Directions for the crust
1. In a medium saucepan, bring the milk to a simmer with the vanilla, sugar, salt, and corn. Cook 5 minutes.
2. While whisking, sprinkle the polenta into the milk.
3. Continue whisking and simmer another 5 minutes.
4. Spray a gratin dish (about 6x8 inch), tart pan, or cake pan with nonstick spray.
5. Pour the polenta into the prepared dish and spread evenly.

### Directions for the filling
1. In a food processor, add the tofu, pumpkin, cream cheese, ginger, syrup, and salt. Mix until smooth.
2. Pour onto the polenta base and fill to the rim of the dish.
3. Bake in 340°F oven about 20 minutes until custard is set.
4. Allow to cool and serve.

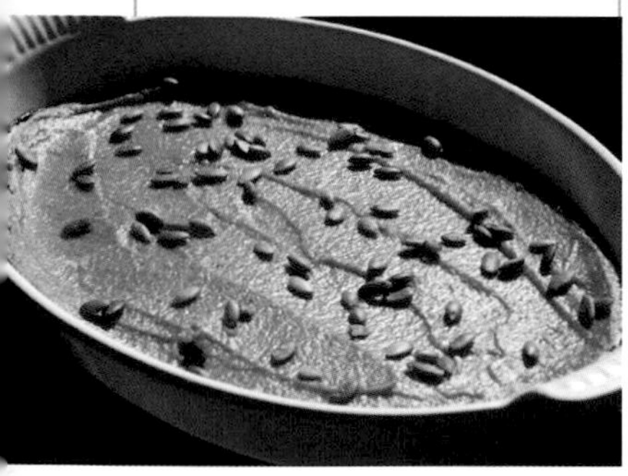

***Notes*** • *To help spread the polenta in the dish, dip a spatula in warm water so the polenta doesn't stick to it. Dip in water as often as needed.* • *If fresh corn is not available, frozen corn also works.*

**Serves 8**
**Nutritional information per serving**
Calories 227
Protein 44g
Carbohydrates 3g
Fat 2g

# Banana Pumpkin Tart

### Ingredients for the dough

2 cups all-purpose flour
⅓ cup water
2 Tbsp butter
1 egg yolk
¼ tsp salt

### Ingredients for the tart filling

1 (8 oz) can pumpkin mix
2 Tbsp nonfat sour cream
½ tsp vanilla extract
3 Tbsp brown sugar
3 bananas (peeled and cut into ⅓-inch pieces)
Grand Marnier or other orange liqueur

### Directions for the dough

1. Preheat oven to 400°F.
2. Place the butter in a glass or plastic dish and microwave until it is melted.
3. In a bowl, combine the flour, egg yolk, water, salt, and butter.
4. By hand or with a plastic bowl scraper, fold the ingredients into the flour.
5. When homogenized, form the dough into a circle about 1 inch thick and 6 inches in diameter.
6. Wrap in plastic wrap, and let rest in the refrigerator for 30 minutes.

### Directions for the filling

1. In a bowl, mix the pumpkin, sour cream, vanilla, and brown sugar.
2. In another small bowl, soak the bananas in Grand Marnier.

### Directions for assembly and baking

1. Roll out the dough on a flat surface with a rolling pin, making sure the table and the dough are dusted with flour. Roll to 12 inches diameter or large enough to fit on a pizza stone.
2. Dust with flour and roll the dough around the rolling pin lightly. Do not apply pressure or the dough will stick. Place on a preheated pizza stone.
3. With a ladle, spread the pumpkin mix and place the pieces of banana on top of the mix.
4. Bake about 20 minutes or until golden brown.
5. Remove the stone and place on a heat-resistant surface.
6. Serve warm or at room temperature.

**Notes** • *Work the dough until it's homogenous. Do not overwork it, or it will shrink when you roll it out.* • *It takes more time for the tart to cook in a tart pan. A hot pizza stone shortens the cooking time.* • *Once the tart is cooked, there won't be any traces of alcohol from soaking the banana in the Grand Marnier or orange liqueur, but there will be a lingering, delicate orange flavor.*

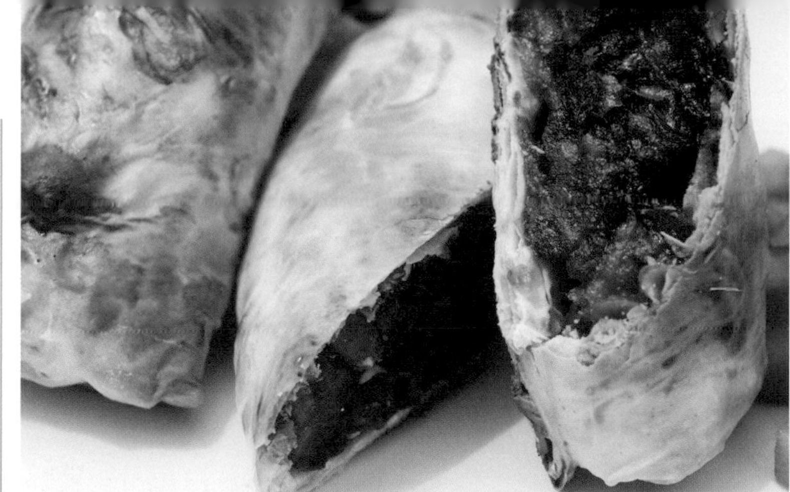

# Banana with Dates in Filo Dough

***Serves 8***
***Nutritional information per serving***
Calories 264
Protein 4g
Carbohydrates 65g
Fat 2g

## Ingredients

- 1 lb bananas (peeled and cut into ½-inch slices)
- ½ cup brown sugar
- 1 tsp vanilla extract
- ⅛ tsp nutmeg
- ¾ cup pitted dry Medjool dates
- ½ package filo dough (defrosted for 24 hours in the refrigerator)
- 1 egg (beaten with a fork and a pinch of salt)
- 4 Tbsp honey
- 1 tsp sesame seeds

## Directions

1. In a heavy-bottom pan, add the banana, brown sugar, vanilla, nutmeg, and dates.
2. Cook slowly, stirring frequently, for 30–45 minutes or until golden brown.
3. Allow to cool.
4. Place a sheet of filo on a cutting board.
5. Brush lightly with beaten egg and sprinkle with ¼ tsp of the sesame seeds.
6. Place another sheet on top of the first one.
7. Follow the same procedure two more times. You should have about 3 or 4 sheets of filo.
8. Cut this stack into 4 rectangles.
9. Place about 2 Tbsp of the banana-date mixture on the center of each stack. Roll into a burrito shape, making sure the ends are tucked in prior to rolling.
10. Brush the top with the egg wash.
11. Bake on a nonstick cookie sheet in a 350°F oven for 8–10 minutes or until golden brown.
12. Let cool.
13. Drizzle with honey and serve.

***Notes*** • *Once the sheets of filo have been unrolled, it is important to cover them with a damp towel. Remove one or two sheets at a time and work quickly before it becomes brittle.* • *Using a heavy-bottom pan allows the banana to cook with less risk of burning.* • *The beaten eggs brushed on pastry before cooking is called an "egg wash."*

# Fig and Greek Yogurt on Golden Granola

***Serves about 8***
***Nutritional information per serving***
Calories 420
Protein 10g
Carbohydrates 65g
Fat 14g

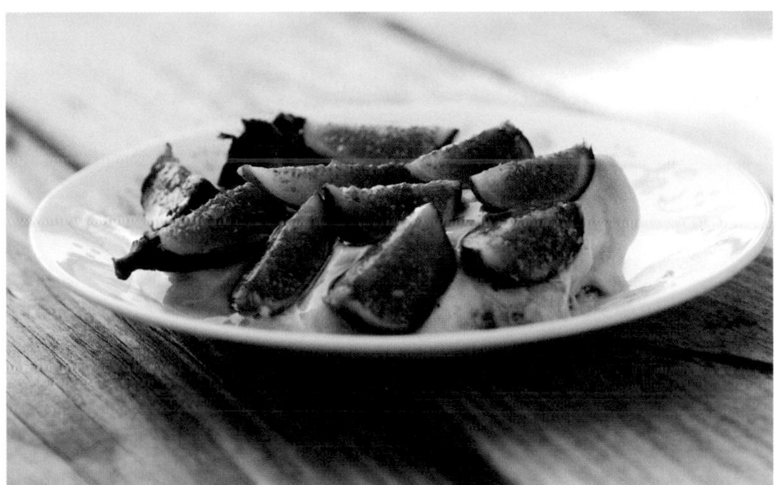

### Ingredients for the crust

3 cups oats
½ cup pecans (cut into ⅛-inch pieces)
½ cup corn syrup
½ cup brown sugar
¼ cup water
3 Tbsp olive oil
¼ tsp salt

### Ingredients for the filling

1 pint figs
1 cup Greek yogurt (such as Fage)
1 cup tofu, extra firm
2 Tbsp brown sugar
1 tsp rose water (or orange blossom water)
Honey or brown sugar, to taste

### Directions for the crust

1. Preheat oven to 325°F.
2. Spray a 9-inch tart or pie pan with nonstick spray.
3. In a bowl, mix oats and pecans.
4. In a 10-inch nonstick pan, combine the corn syrup, brown sugar, salt, water, and oil.
5. Bring to a boil and add the dry ingredients.
6. Mix thoroughly.
7. With a spatula, spread the mixture evenly in the tart or pie pan.
8. Bake 35–40 minutes at 325°F.
9. When the mix is golden brown, remove from oven and let cool.

### Directions for the filling

1. Mix the yogurt, tofu, sugar, and rose water in a blender.
2. Pour into the 9-inch tart or pie pan and bake until set, approximately 15–20 minutes.
3. Allow to cool.
4. Wash the figs and cut into quarters.
5. Place the figs attractively over the tart.
6. Sprinkle with extra honey or brown sugar, if desired.

**Notes** • *If you don't have rose water, substitute orange blossom water or use about ¼ tsp grated orange zest.* • *Dip a spatula in water before spreading the granola crust on the bottom of the tart pan to prevent the mix from sticking to it.*

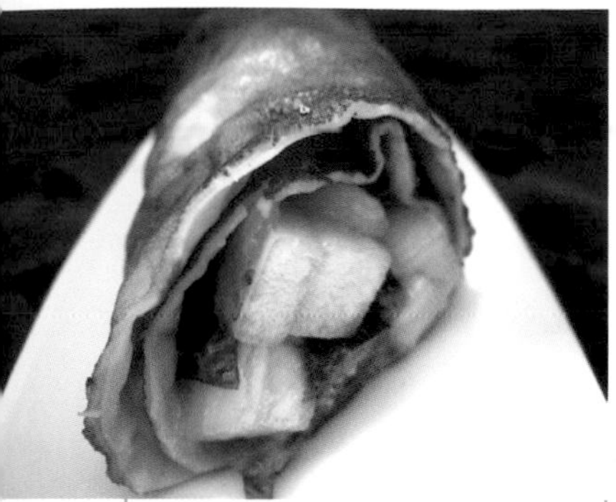

# Honey, Date, Melon, Banana, and Basil Crêpe

***Serves 4 (2 crêpes apiece; makes 8–10)***
***Nutritional information per serving***
Calories 324
Protein 10g
Carbohydrates 65g
Fat 4g

### Ingredients for the crêpes

¾ cup flour
1¼ cup (10 fl oz) milk
2 eggs
Nonstick spray

### Ingredients for the filling

¾ cup dates (pits removed and cut into ⅓-inch pieces)
2 bananas (peeled and cut into ⅓-inch cubes)
1 cup (8 oz) honeydew (skin and seeds removed, cut into ⅓-inch pieces)
6 leaves basil (washed, dried, and sliced thin with a very sharp knife)
1 Tbsp honey

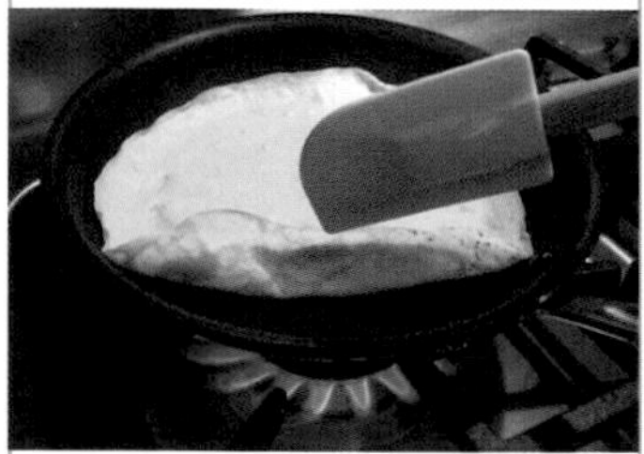

### Directions for the crêpes

1. Place the flour in a large bowl.
2. In a smaller bowl, mix the milk and the eggs.
3. With a whisk, make a well in the middle of the flour for the egg and milk mixture. Add a third of the mixture, and whisk in small circles in the middle of the bowl until it is a thick paste.
4. Work only in the center of the flour. Avoid touching the sides of the bowl, or too much flour will be incorporated and make the batter lumpy.
5. When the batter resembles thick pancake batter, add another third of the milk and whisk until the batter is thinner, with no lumps.
6. Add the last third of the milk and whisk until smooth. If there are still lumps, strain the batter through a fine strainer.

### Cooking the crêpes

1. Heat an 8-inch nonstick pan over medium-low heat.
2. Spray with nonstick spray and wipe off the excess with a paper towel.
3. Use a 2-oz ladle to swirl about the crêpe batter in a very thin layer over the entire bottom of the pan. There should be no excess batter in the pan.
4. Cook until the bottom of the crêpe is golden brown. If it browns too fast, lower the temperature.
5. Flip with a spatula and cook another 30 seconds.
6. Place the crêpe on a plate and repeat the steps until all the batter is used, approximately 8–10 crêpes.

### Directions for the filling

In a bowl, mix the dates, banana, honeydew, and basil. Use immediately.

### Assembling the crêpes

1. Place the crêpe on a flat work surface with the lighter side up.
2. Pour 5 Tbsp of the fruit mix across the center of the crêpe.
3. Fold the right and left edges of the crêpe over toward the middle.
4. Roll the crêpe (similar to rolling a burrito).
5. Serve with a drizzle of honey.

# Ginger Crêpes with Bananas and Cantaloupe

***Serves 4 (2 crêpes apiece)***
***Nutritional information per serving***
Calories 236
Protein 10g
Carbohydrates 41g
Fat 4g

### Ingredients for the crêpes

¾ cup flour
1¼ cup milk (10 fl oz)
2 eggs
Nonstick spray

### Ingredients for the filling

2 ripe bananas (peeled and cut into ½-inch cubes)
½ cantaloupe (skin and seeds removed, diced into ⅓-inch cubes)
1 Tbsp ginger (peeled and grated fine)
2 Tbsp nonfat sour cream

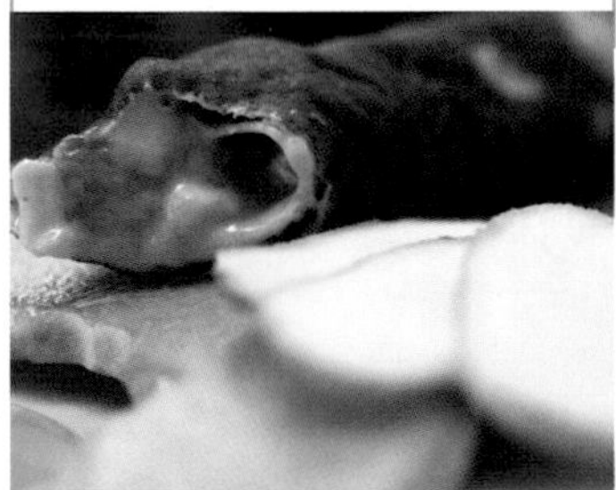

### Directions for the crêpes

1. Place the flour in a large bowl.
2. In a small bowl, mix the milk and the eggs.
3. With a whisk, make a well in the middle of the flour for the egg and milk mixture. Add a third of the mixture, and whisk in small circles in the middle of the bowl until it is a thick paste.
4. Work only in the center of the flour and avoid touching the side of the bowl, or too much flour will be incorporated and the batter will get lumpy.
5. When the batter resembles thick pancake batter, add another third of the milk mixture. Whisk until you achieve a thinner, lump-free batter.
6. Add the last third of the milk, and whisk until smooth. If there are any lumps, strain the batter through a fine strainer.

### Cooking the crêpes

1. Heat an 8-inch nonstick pan over medium-low heat.
2. Spray with nonstick spray and wipe off the excess with a paper towel.
3. Use a 2-oz ladle to swirl the crêpe batter in a very thin layer over the entire bottom of the pan. There should be no loose excess batter in the pan.
4. Cook until the bottom of the crêpe is golden brown. If it's browning too fast, lower the temperature.
5. Flip with a spatula and cook for 30 seconds.
6. Place the crêpe onto a plate and repeat the steps until all the batter is used, approximately 8 crêpes

### Directions for the filling

In a bowl, mix the banana, cantaloupe, ginger, and nonfat sour cream.

### Assembling the crêpes

1. Place the crêpe on a flat work surface with the lighter side up.
2. Pour 5 Tbsp of the fruit mix across the center of the crêpe.
3. Fold over the right and left edges of the crêpe toward the middle.
4. Roll the crêpe (similar to rolling a burrito).

**Notes** • *You can sprinkle the crêpe with confectioner's sugar or a few sprinkles of brown sugar.*

# Tropical Ginger and Aloe Rice Pudding

*Serves 12*
***Nutritional information per serving***
Calories 124
Protein 4g
Carbohydrates 25g
Fat 1g

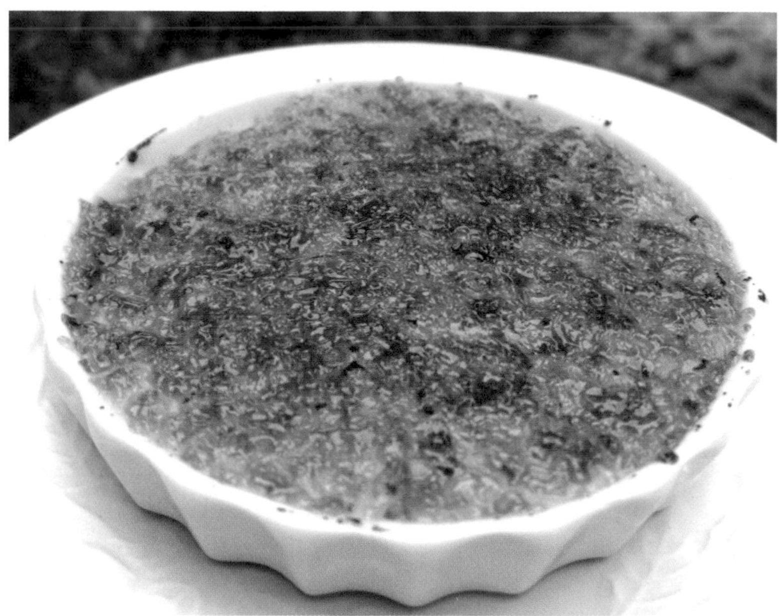

## Ingredients

- 1 cup rice (arborio rice preferred)
- 4¼ cups milk
- 2 tsp ginger (peeled and grated fine)
- 1 egg yolk
- 1 vanilla bean (split in half with a paring knife and scraped)
- ¼ cup brown sugar
- 1 tsp salt
- ⅓ cup fresh aloe vera (skin removed and diced into ¼-inch cubes)
- ½ cup turbinado sugar (turbinado has more of a molasses taste)

## Directions

1. In a medium saucepan, bring the milk to a boil. Add the vanilla bean and scrapings. Lower the heat to simmer.
2. Whisk the ginger and rice into the milk. Cover the saucepan halfway with a lid and simmer for about 25 minutes. Remove from heat.
3. In a bowl, mix the brown sugar, salt, aloe vera, and egg yolk.
4. Immediately pour it into the rice, and mix for about 1 minute.
5. Fill individual crème brulee molds to the rim and allow to cool.
6. Just before serving, sprinkle each dessert with a thin layer of turbinado sugar. Remove the excess sugar by flipping each mold upside down for a second. With a towel, clean the rims completely.
7. With a blowtorch, brown the sugar slightly.

***Notes*** • *If the rice is not cooked enough and begins to stick to the bottom, add ½ cup milk.* • *Make sure the rims of the molds are completely cleaned with the tip of a towel. Any sugar that is left on the rim will burn immediately when it comes in contact with the blowtorch flame.* • *If you don't have a blowtorch or are afraid of using one, bake in a preheated broiler until the sugar begins to caramelize and slightly change color. Remove from oven and serve lukewarm.* • *The egg yolk becomes pasteurized when mixed with the simmering rice. Together, the egg and rice mixture reach a temperature of 180°F.*

# Pear Cardamom Sorbet

*Serves 15*
*Nutritional information per serving*
Calories 153
Protein 2g
Carbohydrates 38g
Fat 0.5g

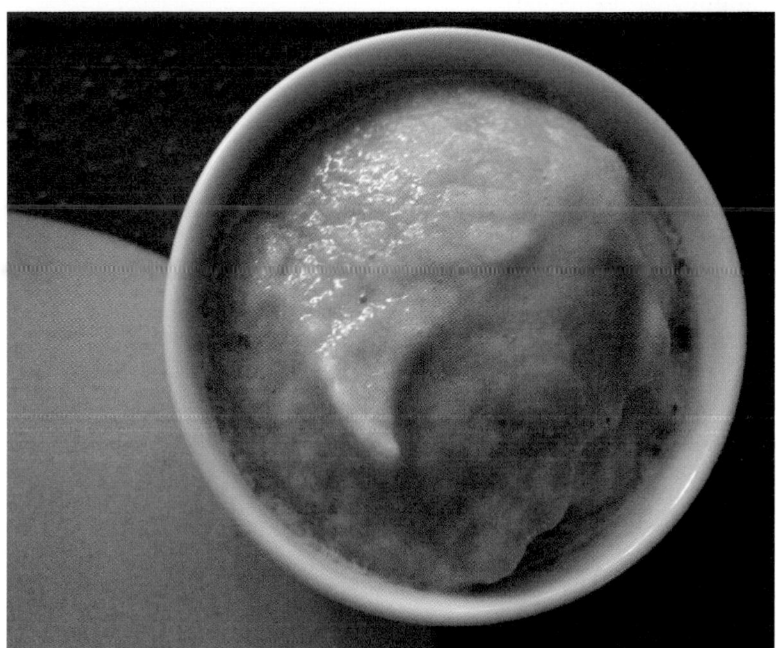

### Ingredients

2 lbs fresh Bartlett pears (washed, peeled, halved, cored, and cut into 1-inch pieces)
3 cups water
1½ cups honey
½ tsp salt
1 tsp vanilla extract
1 tsp grated ginger (peeled and grated fine)
⅛ tsp ground cardamom
2 cups milk

### Directions

1. In a large saucepan, add to water the pears, honey, salt, vanilla, ginger, and cardamom.
2. Bring to a boil and simmer for 20 minutes or until pears are tender.
3. Using a hand blender, mix until smooth.
4. Cool and place in ice cube trays. Freeze overnight.

### To serve

1. Remove the cubes of pear purée from the ice cube trays.
2. Place 1 cup of the milk and ¾ of the pear cubes in the blender. Blend until smooth.
3. Adjust to the desired consistency either by adding the rest of the milk or more pear cubes.

**Notes** • *I like to leave the skin on the pears for the vitamins, but remember to wash the pears thoroughly.* • *Today there are great blenders on the market with incredible power. I use a blender by Vitamix that comes with a tamper, which helps eliminate chunks.* • *If you're using canned pears, make the sorbet the same day. Place the drained pears in a blender and add the honey, salt, vanilla, ginger, cardamom, and ice. Blend and add milk to the desired consistency.* • *Try to use very ripe pears. The pear season in the U.S. is from September to February. A ripe pear turns yellow and bruises easily.*

*Serves 8*
***Nutritional information per serving***
Calories 80
Protein 0.1g
Carbohydrates 23g
Fat 0.1g

# Watermelon and Ginger Granité

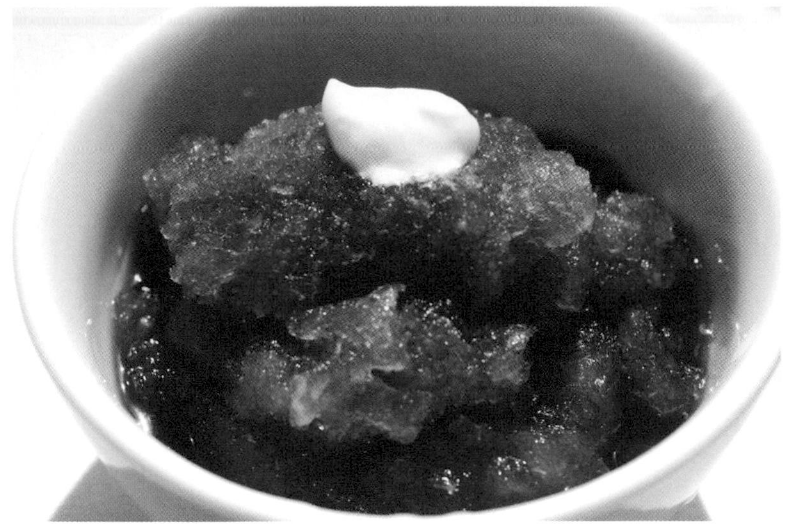

### Ingredients

3 cups seedless watermelon juice (melon cut in half, flesh removed and blended)
1 cup water
½ cup honey
1 whole clove
1 pinch ground nutmeg
1 tsp fresh ginger (peeled and grated fine)
¼ tsp salt
½ tsp lemon zest (washed and grated fine)

### Directions

1. Bring the water, honey, clove, nutmeg, ginger, salt, and lemon zest to a boil. Allow to cool, then strain.
2. Add the mixture to the watermelon juice.
3. Place the juice in a bowl that can be put in the freezer, and freeze 3 hours. Stir every 15 minutes with a sauce whisk.

**Notes** • *The granité can also be left in the freezer overnight and grated with a regular fork. This way, it does not need to be stirred every 15 minutes while freezing.*

*Serves 10*
***Nutritional information per serving***
Calories 45
Protein 0.5g
Carbohydrates 12g
Fat 0.1g

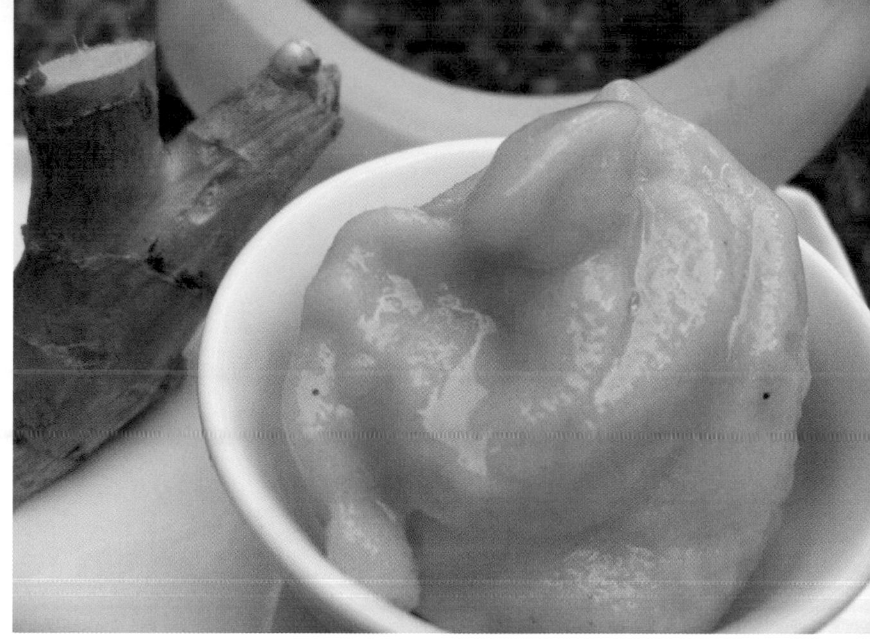

# Quick Banana Sorbet

## Ingredients

3 bananas, peeled
1 Tbsp ginger (peeled and grated fine)
⅛ tsp ground cardamom
2 Tbsp honey
¼ tsp salt
3 cups ice

## Directions

1. Place the bananas, ginger, cardamom, honey, and salt in the blender.
2. Blend on high until smooth.
3. Add ice and blend until creamy. Add more ice as needed.
4. Serve immediately or store in freezer.

***Notes*** • *To make this sorbet, it's best to use a heavy-duty blender with a tamper that allows you to push the ice cubes down toward the blender blades.* • *If an air pocket forms around the blades of the blender, stop the blender, stir, and start again.*

# Butterscotch Praline Mousse

*Serves 8*
*Nutritional information per serving*
Calories 204
Protein 5g
Carbohydrates 36g
Fat 5g

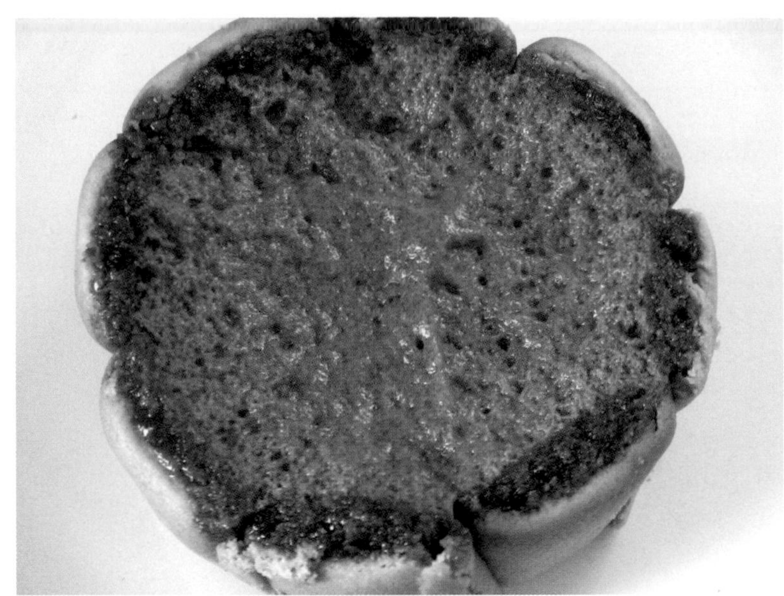

## Ingredients

1 cup sugar
⅓ cup water
3 Tbsp butter
1 tsp gelatin powder (soaked in 3 Tbsp warm water)
4 fl oz milk (keep 1 fl oz cold; bring 3 fl oz to a boil)
1 tsp cornstarch (mix with the 1 fl oz cold milk)
⅓ cup nonfat sour cream
6 egg whites
⅛ tsp salt
1 Tbsp Frangelico liqueur
4 ladyfingers (cut in ½-inch cubes and soaked in the Frangelico)
1 ripe banana (peeled and cut in ½-inch slices)

## Directions

1. Place the water and sugar in a saucepan. Bring to a boil.
2. Stir the pan to swirl the sugar and help it cook evenly.
3. When the sugar is a deep golden brown, add the butter and swirl again. Be very careful, as the caramel is over 260°F.
4. In a bowl, soak the gelatin in the water.
5. In a separate saucepan, bring 3 fl oz of milk to a boil and add the slurry of cornstarch and cold milk. Whisk constantly while bringing to a boil. Add the gelatin, whisk, and allow to cool to room temperature.
6. Add the thick milk to the warm sugar.
7. Cool down while whisking frequently.
8. When room temperature, add the sour cream.
9. In a large bowl, add salt and egg whites. Whisk until soft peaks form.
10. Fold into the milk, sugar, and sour cream mixture. Mix carefully with a rubber spatula.
11. Spoon into individual martini glasses, layering the cream with a few cubes of lightly soaked ladyfingers and bananas.
12. Refrigerate 2 hours and serve cold.
13. Optional: garnish with fruits of your choice.

# Sweet Potato and Cantaloupe Cake

***Serves 10***
***Nutritional information per serving***
Calories 205
Protein 4g
Carbohydrates 45g
Fat 2g

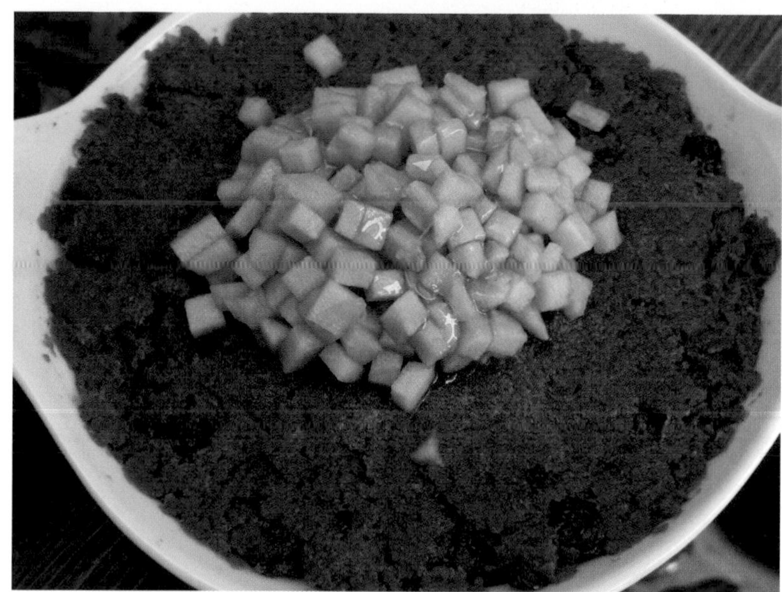

## Ingredients

2 lbs sweet potato (peeled and grated coarse)
1 Tbsp fine-grated ginger
2 ripe bananas (peeled and cut in ½-inch sections)
4 Tbsp brown sugar
4 Tbsp raisins
¼ tsp salt
½ tsp vanilla extract
2 Tbsp rum
½ tsp ground nutmeg
⅛ tsp ground clove
1 Tbsp lime zest
½ cup sweet condensed milk
1 cantaloupe (cut in half, seeds and skin removed, and cut into ¼-inch pieces)
Honey or agave nectar, to taste

## Directions

1. In a heavy-bottomed pan, add the sweet potato, ginger, banana, sugar, raisins, salt, vanilla, rum, nutmeg, cloves, lime zest, and milk.
2. Cook slowly, stirring often with a wooden spoon, 40–60 minutes.
3. Place in a tart pan coated with nonstick pan spray.
4. Spread the mix and let cool.
5. Cover with cantaloupe and drizzle with honey or agave nectar to taste.
6. Serve promptly or refrigerate.

***Notes*** • *There is no alcohol in the dessert. The alcohol evaporates during cooking, leaving a rum flavor that adds to the complexity of the taste.*

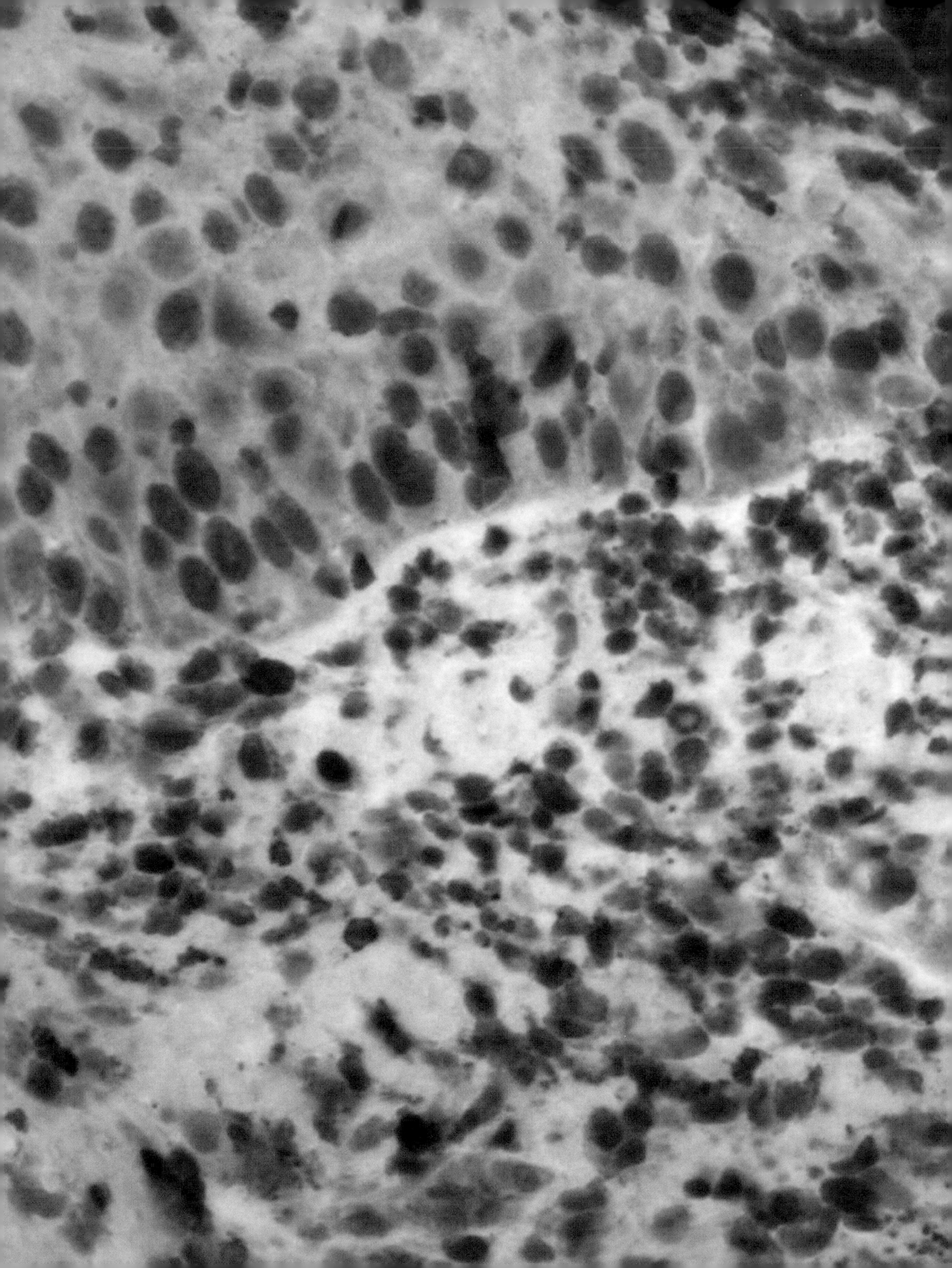

# *the* science

# Reflux Science You Can Digest

Jamie A. Koufman, M.D., F.A.C.S.

**re·flux** *n* [ L *re-* back + *fluxus* flow ] 1: a flowing back 2: a process of refluxing

This may come as a surprise, but reflux is more complicated and controversial than almost any other common disease.[1-3] Reflux is like the elephant in the famous tale of the three blind men and the elephant:

> *The first blind man, feeling the leg of the elephant, exclaims, "I can see it clearly; the elephant is like a tree." The second blind man holds the trunk and says, "No, the elephant is like a very large snake." The third blind man grasps an ear. "Aha, you are both wrong," he says. "The elephant is rather like a giant leaf." Each of the blind men embraces a part of the truth, but none understands its entirety.*

In this chapter, I will attempt to describe the whole elephant, drawing in large measure from my almost thirty years of basic scientific and clinical research into reflux disease.[1-59]

In the case of reflux, the three blind men might be represented by three medical specialties, each one focusing on a different part of the aerodigestive tract: (1) The *otolaryngologist* (ENT physician) specializes in the ears, nose, and throat; (2) the *gastroenterologist* (GI physician) specializes in the esophagus (the swallowing tube that connects the throat with the stomach); and (3) the *pulmonologist* (PUL physician) specializes in the lungs. Many other medical specialties encounter patients with reflux as well, including internists, family practitioners, pediatricians, and critical care specialists.

Reflux remains controversial. Part of the problem is that each medical specialty has its own language and set of diseases related to reflux. While "acid reflux" is the most common lay term for the disease, GERD and LPR are the terms widely used by GIs and ENTs, respectively. See Table 1 for a list of common terms for reflux. That there are so many different terms for reflux suggests fragmentation within the medical community with regard to the mechanisms and manifestations of disease. To make matters worse, most medical specialists remain unaware of the literature and research from other specialties. At least the three blind men in the fable shared their findings with each other—because medical specialists don't.

**Table 1**
**MOST COMMON MEDICAL TERMS FOR REFLUX**

| |
|---|
| Gastroesophageal reflux disease (GERD) |
| Gastro-oesophageal reflux disease (GORD) |
| Reflux esophagitis, esophageal erosions |
| Extraesophageal reflux disease |
| Supraesophageal reflux disease |
| Atypical reflux disease |
| Laryngopharyngeal reflux (LPR) |
| Silent reflux |

## The History of Reflux

In its most elemental form, reflux is the backflow of gastric (stomach) contents into the esophagus (the muscular swallowing tube between the throat and stomach). The term for this is gastroesophageal reflux. Reflux was not actually described until the twentieth century, but severe burning chest pain after eating, known as heartburn, was recognized in antiquity as a predictable outcome of gluttony.[1]

Reflux as a disease was first reported in 1935 by Winkelstein,[60] who described "peptic ulcer of the esophagus." He postulated that the esophageal injury was due to the backflow of the contents from the stomach. Prior to that, physicians had recognized diseases of the esophagus such as erosions, inflammation, and stricture (narrowing because of scarring), along with the symptom heartburn. However, they believed that those esophageal findings were attributable to diseases such as tuberculosis and gall stones.[1]

In the 1940s and 1950s, x-ray imaging of the esophagus became popular (using the barium swallow), and the finding of a hiatal hernia became synonymous with a diagnosis of gastroesophageal reflux disease (hiatal hernia is the name for an anatomic finding seen during a barium swallow; it is a kind of deformity of the stomach valve, known as the lower esophageal sphincter, in which the uppermost portion of the stomach slides upward into the chest).

At that time, the only effective antireflux medication was Tagamet (an H2-antagonist, similar to today's Zantac), and for a person with severe heartburn and a hiatal hernia, antireflux surgery was often recommended.[61,62] We now know that it isn't that simple; that is, people can have reflux without a hiatal hernia, and people can have a hiatal hernia without having reflux. What is true is that many people with reflux do have such a hernia, which implies a relatively weak lower esophageal valve. However, the presence of a hiatal hernia is not an indication for surgery. Today, laparoscopic antireflux surgery ("fundoplication") is still the treatment of choice for many patients with severe or recalcitrant reflux, especially LPR.[41,62,63]

In the 1960s and 1970s, clinical (diagnostic) technology matured, including the growing use of esophageal manometry (to assess and measure swallowing and esophageal function),[64,65] flexible endoscopes and endoscopy,[66] and pH (acid) monitoring systems.[67-69] With these diagnostics and some new treatments, a better understanding of managing GERD began to emerge.[70-87] LPR, however, was still in the shadows.

Meanwhile, remember those three blind men? It is worthwhile to consider the history of reflux in terms of who discovered what and when. The fragmentation of the understanding of reflux as a disease is in large measure because of turf battles in academic medicine and ignorance of the research from other specialties.

In recent history, otolaryngology (ENT) and gastroenterology (GI) have been sharing the reflux pie, but the father of modern endoscopy was an ENT surgeon named Chevalier Jackson.[88] In 1890, Jackson invented the distal-lighted esophagoscope—a hollow, rigid metal instrument for examining the esophagus.[1] For most of the twentieth century, Jackson and his disciples in ENT were the ones performing endoscopy of the breathing and digestive passages.

In the late 1960s, with invention of the flexible endoscope,[66] many of the specialists in gastroesophageal reflux disease (GERD) became gastroenterologists.

In the early 1980s, there was cooperation and collaboration between GIs and ENTs,[3,5-7] but with the discovery of laryngopharyngeal reflux (LPR), reflux into the larynx (voice box) and pharynx (throat), and with the advent of transnasal esophagoscopy[24,33,45,58,89,90] (TNE), cooperation broke down. The problem was one of perception—each group witnessed different reflux manifestations and syndromes in their patients.

## LPR Is Different Than GERD

Many reflux patients are frustrated because their doctors only understand classical GERD, so if their symptoms differ, they're out of luck. While I was writing this book, I gave a preview chapter to a patient who shared it with her local doctor. She then reported to me that her local doctor insisted that her barium swallow showed no signs of reflux, and, that my chapter was "a lot of bunk." "But he didn't even read it," she said. I tell this story here to emphasize that there is still a wide schism between specialties.

Prior to my work on LPR (silent reflux), there were a few brave pioneers who suggested that reflux was not just GERD;[91-100] however, the literature on it was sparse and most of the reports anecdotal. Some of those who deserve credit for seminal thinking on LPR and who most influenced me were Nels Olson,[96] Don Cherry,[91] Paul Ward,[100] Paul Chodosh,[94] and Bob Toohill.[101] I remember Dr. Olson warning me that LPR was a hot potato subject, and that some of his academic contemporaries had tried to discredit him over his belief that LPR was ubiquitous and caused a myriad of airway diseases. Of course, when Dr. Olson talked about reflux, he referred to it as GERD. In the past two decades, there have been many reports linking reflux to diseases of the ears, nose, throat, and lungs.[95-124]

In 1991, the year my Triological Society thesis was published,[1] I coined the term *laryngopharyngeal reflux*. I felt we needed a new way to describe the type of "silent" reflux seen in many of our patients. I chose that particular term to call attention to how the symptoms and manifestations were laryngeal and pharyngeal, not esophageal. I also believed that the diagnosis and treatment of LPR were different than for GERD. The idea was to intentionally create a nosological distinction between the specialties so that ENT physicians would consider ideas that did not yet have credibility among GI colleagues.

Incidentally, it was Dr. Walter Bo, chair of the anatomy department at Wake

Forest University, who first uttered the term "silent reflux." In 1988, Walter was my patient. After I explained how one could have reflux without also having heartburn, he rolled his eyes and said, "I get it. I have the silent kind of reflux." "Yes, Walter," I said. "That's it; you have SILENT REFLUX."

Although I was trained as an ENT (ear, nose, and throat) doctor, I began limiting my practice to laryngology (voice, throat, and swallowing disorders) in 1981, the same year I began noticing patients with laryngeal manifestations of reflux without heartburn. At the time, I was at Wake Forest University, and I went to gastroenterologists there to discuss my patients.

The head of the department was initially skeptical that reflux could actually affect the larynx. So I convinced one of his fellows to help me study my patients with hoarseness using pH devices that were available for monitoring GERD in the GI department.

In 1984, we began to study patients with laryngeal inflammation, whether or not they had GI symptoms; most of them didn't. The patients actually wore two separate pH monitors—small, soft catheters, one of which went into the esophagus, the other into the throat. Both tubes were connected to minicomputers that continuously measured acidity. The computers recorded any reflux events that occurred and stored the information for subsequent analysis.

Thus was born ambulatory 24-hour double-probe (simultaneous pharyngeal and esophageal) pH monitoring.

We reported our first pH testing results in 1986.[5] Yes, the patients with hoarseness had refluxed into the throat. By 1987, I had my own reflux-testing laboratory, and we were beginning to accumulate data suggesting that LPR patients typically had reflux patterns that were qualitatively and quantitatively different from patients with classic GERD.[1,6,7,15,17]

Sadly even today, quality reflux testing is only performed in a few places. At the Voice Institute of New York, we routinely employ complete high-definition manometry, ambulatory (simultaneous pharyngeal and esophageal) pH monitoring with ISFET technology and new software that analyzes the data at every pH level,[3] and transnasal esophagoscopy. This combination of technologies defines the patterns, mechanisms, and severity of disease so that treatment can be customized for each patient. That is the state of the art.

By 1989, we already understood that the mechanisms and patterns of reflux in LPR were different than those of GERD.[1,3-7,23,27,33] Most GERD patients had heartburn, esophagitis, dysmotility, and a supine (nocturnal) reflux pattern with prolonged periods of acid/pepsin exposure.[1-3,5-7,10,17,27,32,33] Conversely, LPR patients usually did not have heartburn or esophagitis, and an upright (daytime) reflux pattern predominated.[1-3,5-7,32,33] A summary of the typical differences between LPR and GERD is shown below.

### Table 2
### SUMMARY OF THE TYPICAL DIFFERENCES BETWEEN GERD & LPR

| | GERD | LPR |
|---|---|---|
| **Symptoms** | | |
| Heartburn and/or regurgitation | ++++ | + |
| Hoarseness, cough, dysphagia, globus | + | ++++ |
| **Findings** | | |
| Heartburn and/or regurgitation | ++++ | + |
| Hoarseness, cough, dysphagia, globus | + | ++++ |
| **Test Results** | | |
| Erosive esophagitis or Barrett's | +++ | + |
| Abnormal esophageal pH monitoring | ++++ | ++ |
| Abnormal pharyngeal pH monitoring | + | ++++ |
| Esophageal dysmotility | +++ | + |
| Abnormal esophageal acid clearance | ++++ | + |
| **Pattern of Reflux** | | |
| Supine (nocturnal) reflux | ++++ | + |
| Upright (daytime) reflux | + | ++++ |
| Both (abnormal upright and supine reflux) | + | +++ |
| **Response to Treatment** | | |
| Effectiveness of dietary and lifestyle modifications | ++ | + |
| Successful treatment with single-dose PPIs* | +++ | + |
| Successful treatment with twice-daily PPIs | ++++ | +++ |

*PPIs = Proton pump inhibitors (such as Nexium, Protonix, Prilosec, Prevacid, and Zegerid)*

## Pepsin, Not Acid, Causes Reflux Disease (LPR and GERD)

One of the key differences between LPR and GERD is that the thresholds for laryngeal and esophageal damage are quite different.[1,39,42,49] Based on normative pH monitoring data, one can have up to fifty esophageal reflux (pH <4) events, occurring mostly after meals, and that is considered normal. In the larynx, as few as three episodes a week may be too many.[1] In addition, pepsin, and not acid, is the primary injurious component of the refluxate.[1,28,39,125-128] From animal experiments, we know that acid and pepsin in combination (i.e., activated pepsin) produces more tissue damage than any other combination of enzymes. Adding bile salts to the mix, for example, reduces the potency of the refluxate.[1,127,128]

The GI and ENT literature both agree that it is pepsin and not acid that produces tissue damage.[1,127,128] Unfortunately, some of the GI literature suggests that pepsin is inactive above pH 4; however, those experiments were done using pig pepsin.[126] Our laboratory has unequivocally demonstrated that human pepsin is active up to pH 6.[54] See the pepsin activity curve in "What You Eat Could Be Eating You," page 24.

Most of the important bench research including reflux-related cell biology was performed in my laboratory at Wake Forest University and with collaborators in the United Kingdom.[28,39,42,47-49,51,53-57] The papers were reported in prestigious, peer-reviewed medical journals, yet it would seem that this robust scientific literature has gone largely unnoticed outside the specialty of ENT.

Here is a summation of the most important findings and their implications for understanding reflux disease:

- Pepsin, the main digestive enzyme of the stomach, can attach (bind) to tissue and destroy protein, gain access to the cell, and disrupt normal cellular function.[39,42,48,49,53-55,124,129]
- Pepsin requires some acid for its activation, and human pepsin is active across the pH range from 1–6, with 100 percent activity at pH 2 and 10 percent activity at pH 6.[54]
- Patients with reflux laryngitis (LPR) have pepsin on and within their laryngeal tissue, and that pepsin can remain attached for a long time, which may be reactivated by acid from any source, including acidic foods and beverages.[42]

- In studies to date, the tissue-damage protein profiles for reflux laryngitis and for laryngeal cancer are similar;[3,39] see Table 4.
- Reflux is associated with the development of Barrett's Esophagus, a precursor of esophageal cancer; it occurs as frequently in patients with LPR symptoms as it does in patients with classical GERD.[131-135]
- Clinically, patients with reflux symptoms improve when the amount of acid in the diet is limited.[136] Dr. Koufman reported results of a clinical trial of a series of patients with recalcitrant LPR. (Recalcitrant was defined as failed treatment on high-dose antireflux medicines.) These patients were treated with the **Induction Reflux Diet** (nothing below pH 5) for a minimum of two weeks; 95 percent improved significantly, and notably some became completely symptom free.[136]
- Finally, the prevalence of all forms of reflux is increasing, especially among the younger population in the United States.[137]

## Integrated Aerodigestive Medicine

In attempting to describe the whole elephant, I must reiterate that the three blind men exemplify the fragmentation of the medical community. In 2009, I spoke on "Specialization: When Being the Best Isn't Good Enough," in a presidential address to the American Broncho-Esophagological Association. In that speech, I urged that the specialties of otolaryngology, gastroenterology, and pulmonology might be merged to form a new "specialty," *Integrated Aerodigestive Medicine.* The problem with specialists, I argued, is that they only know about a defined anatomic zone; however, reflux is a disease of the entire aerodigestive tract, the components of which are shown in the Table 3.

These anatomic zones are all connected to each other, and it is preposterous to presume that reflux disease respects the boundaries of our medical specialties. It is puzzling, for example, why pulmonary doctors have been slow to embrace reflux as an important cause of pulmonary disease.[8,15,106,107] In my opinion, LPR is responsible for up to 70 percent of lung disease.

I am an expert on LPR and silent reflux. I actually coined both terms. I recognize, however, that I am still one of the blind men in spite of my desire to take care of whole patients. This work points to the urgent need for collaborative research, particularly in translational cell biology that crosses specialty lines.

In a later section of this chapter, "The Missing Link," you will see that there is another gaping hole in our knowledge: We know almost nothing about environmental medicine and about the health risks of what we eat. I fear that within our lifetimes we have all been part of an appalling scientific experiment in which unintended and unforeseen consequences of well-intentioned scientists—whose focus was to make food safe from bacterial contamination—might have led us to a national public health crisis. Reflux is ubiquitous, and its consequences are serious, even deadly.

**Table 3**
**COMPONENTS OF THE AERODIGESTIVE TRACT**

**Nose and sinuses**
**Mouth (oral cavity)**
**Throat (pharynx)**
**Voice box (larynx)**
**Swallowing tube (esophagus)**
**Stomach and upper intestines**
**Breathing tube (trachea) and lungs**

## Reflux and Cancer

One of the most frequent questions patients ask is whether reflux can cause cancer. I believe the answer is an emphatic yes. That is part of the reason this book is so concerned about the acidity of today's typical diet.

We have not yet proven that reflux causes laryngeal and vocal cord cancer, but there is strong circumstantial clinical evidence along with bench research to support it.[1,7,9,39,114,119-124] We believe that one can get laryngeal cancer without smoking, but not without the presence of reflux.[4,39] This section presents six arguments to support this concept.

1. **Many patients with laryngeal cancer are nonsmokers or ex-smokers.** We prospectively studied fifty adult patients with early vocal cord cancer.[9] Of them, 44 percent (22/50) were active smokers, 42 percent (21/50) were ex-smokers with a median duration of smoking cessation of eight years, and 14 percent

(7/50) were lifetime nonsmokers. Using pH monitoring, we found that 68 percent of the patients had reflux, almost twice as many as those who were actually smokers. And remember, in the study group, there were seven lifetime nonsmokers.[9]

2. **Some people get recurrent, small, reflux-related vocal cord cancers that are periodically removed with a surgical laser.** We've seen many such cases over the years. Significantly, almost half of those patients stop making cancer when their reflux is controlled. The same is true for patients with precancers called dysplasia and leukoplakia.[1,114]
3. **When different groups of patients are tested for reflux, including those with cough, sore throat, etc., the highest proportion of those demonstrating reflux are the cancer patients.** In 1991, we reported abnormal reflux testing in 84 percent (21/25) of patients with laryngeal cancer, five of whom were lifetime nonsmokers.[1]
4. **We compared the reflux (pH) testing results of smokers and nonsmokers and found that smokers had twice as much reflux, both in the esophagus and the throat.** Cigarette smoking is specifically associated with relaxation of the upper and lower esophageal valves within two minutes, and reflux episodes occur with two-thirds of cigarettes smoked.[55,138]
5. **Our laboratory has examined the impact of reflux on a cellular level in human patients and in animal models and found tremendous similarities in the larynx between patients who have LPR and patients who have cancer.** Of those studies, the most important was an analysis of biopsies for the presence of pepsin within the laryngeal tissue. Pepsin was found in 5 percent (1/20) of normal controls without reflux. On the other hand, 95 percent of LPR patients with reflux into the throat had pepsin in their laryngeal biopsy tissue, and 100 percent (5/5) of laryngeal cancer patients tested had pepsin within the cancerous tissue.[39,47,55] In addition, extraordinary landmark experiments in cell biology by Nikki Johnston *et al.* [42,47,48,51.53,54,124] showed that pepsin up-regulates the genes that cause cancer in a way that suggests that pepsin is actually the cause of laryngeal cancer.[124]
6. **There are similarities between laryngeal cancer and esophageal cancer.** **Figure 1** below shows the presence of pepsin in reflux laryngitis by a special staining technique (**Figure 1A**), and within a Barrett's Esophagus biopsy specimen (**Figure 1B**).

## Figure 1: PEPSIN IMMUNOCHEMISTRY (IHC)

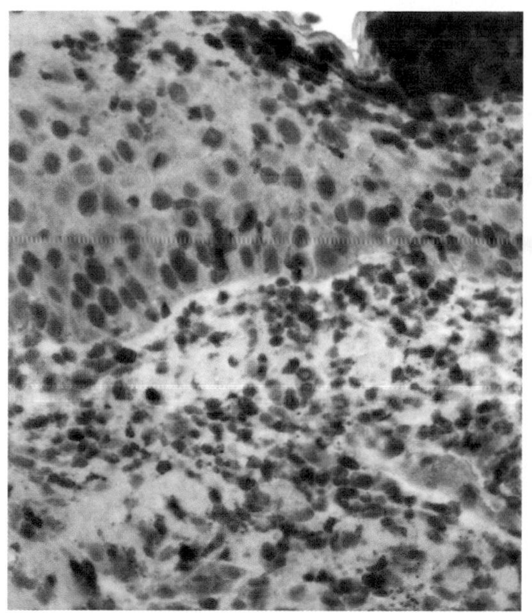

**A.** Reflux laryngitis showing pepsin by IHC

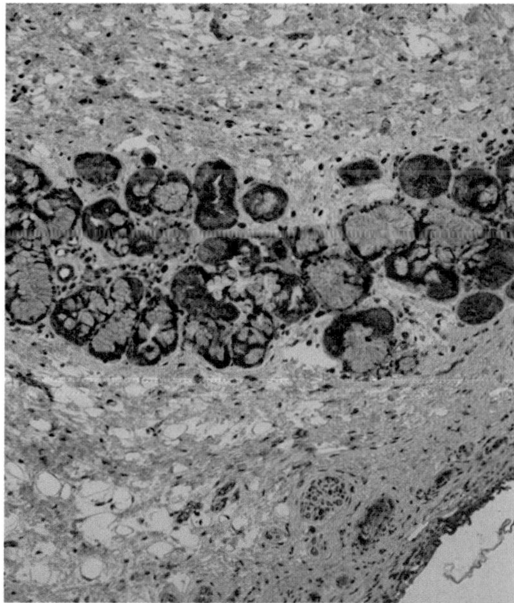

**B.** Pepsin in Barrett's Esophagus by IHC

The table below summarizes the cell biology findings. As you can see, reflux and laryngeal cancer have the same protein profiles except for one stress protein, HSP70.[4,39,47-49]

Table 4
**TISSUE PROFILE OF LPR, CARCINOMA, AND CONTROLS**

| | Controls | LPR | Cancer |
|---|---|---|---|
| Pepsin | None | + | + |
| CAIII | ☒ | ☒ | ☒ |
| E-Cadherin | ☒ | ☒ | ☒ |
| SEP70 | ☒ | ☒ | ☒ |
| SEP53 | ☒ | ☒ | ☒ |
| HSP70 | ☒ | ☒ | ☒ |

+ = Positive (present)
☒ = Normal (baseline) level
☒ = Decreased compared to normal controls

As previously mentioned, esophageal cancer is one of the fastest-growing cancers in the United States, and we are finding Barrett's Esophagus, a known reflux-related form of precancer, in approximately 7 percent of our LPR reflux patients.[33,44,52] It is striking and significant to note that Barrett's Esophagus is found just as often in ENT patients with silent reflux (symptoms of coughing and hoarseness) as in GI patients with heartburn.[134]

In summary, there is clinical and scientific evidence that reflux, mainly pepsin, may cause cancer of the larynx and esophagus.

The brown material in biopsy specimens shown in **Figure 1A** and **1B** is pepsin stained by a special technique. It's easy to see how dietary acid from above could stimulate that pepsin the same way as could acid from below.

One of our biggest concerns is that a huge population of Americans is potentially at risk to develop cancer, and that we have no methodology for identifying the most susceptible. As clinicians, we can certainly say that we are seeing increasingly more and more reflux in increasingly younger patients; and this in our opinion, is an ominous warning sign.

We recognize that we may be criticized as alarmists, and we regret that we cannot prove all of our assertions and beliefs just yet. However, our data and clinical impressions deserve to be in the public domain so that other researchers and clinicians can investigate the relationships we've presented. We believe that diet is the missing link and that our diet may be killing us, and it is time for us to aggressively explore these variables and fix them.

By the way, people who are rightfully worried about cancer deserve to be checked. The technology has changed. Doctors can now look inside while patients are awake, comfortable, and without pain, using a technique called transnasal esophagoscopy.[29,33,58,134] The idea that you can only be checked for cancer in a special facility and under anesthesia is archaic.

## The Missing Link

Why is reflux epidemic? Why is esophageal cancer one of the fastest-growing cancers in America? Why are so many people with reflux failing medical treatment? We believe that the answer is related to high levels of dietary acid. How and when did this happen?

While this story of the reflux epidemic focuses on acid, we should point out that since WWII there have been four significant dietary trends. Counting the increased acidification of prepared foods and beverages, they are: Increased saturated fat; increased sugar (low-glycemic index carbs); and increased use of preservatives, stabilizers, thickeners, and artificial sweeteners. Here's the story.

**Table 5**
**LANDMARKS AND MILESTONES IN THE AMERICAN DIET**

| | |
|---|---|
| 1886 | Coca-Cola invented; Pepsi-Cola invented in 1893 |
| 1919 | American Bottlers of Carbonated Beverages formed |
| 1952 | First diet soda pop sold (Kirsch No-Cal Ginger Ale) |
| 1955 | McDonald's Corporation formed; fast food is born |
| 1962 | Instant foods become common in American homes |
| 1963 | McDonald's begins marketing meals for families |
| 1965 | Canned soda first distributed in vending machines |
| 1966 | The National Soft Drink Association is formed |
| 1967 | High-fructose corn syrup is introduced |
| 1973 | Title 21: Law is in response to outbreak of botulism |
| 1985 | "New Coke" introduced with high-fructose syrup |
| 1990 | Nutrition Labeling and Information Act passed |
| 2003 | Report: Junk food represents ⅓ of American calories |

## How and When the American Diet Changed

Coca-Cola was invented in 1886 by a pharmacist in Atlanta, and Pepsi-Cola came along a few years later.[140] These were fountain drinks and weren't actually bottled until the twentieth century. Coca-Cola rose to prominence as America's drink during and after WWII. While the recipe and ingredients have changed over the years, this drink and others like it have always been very acidic. The current pH (acidity) of Coca-Cola is 2.8, as acidic as stomach acid itself.

The American Bottlers of Carbonated Beverages was formed in 1919. After many years and a few name changes, they became a national lobby.

The first diet soda pop made its debut in 1952. This represented a new potential market for the soda industry, but it also introduced a host of additives and chemicals. Today, some diet drinks are more acidic than their nondiet counterparts.

In 1955, Roy Kroc started the McDonald's Corporation. Most baby boomers can remember when they first encountered McDonald's. (Personally, I recall buying a hamburger in Dedham, Massachusetts, in the early 1960s for nineteen cents.)

By 1962, instant foods, such as instant milk and instant pudding, were common in almost every American household. These products were essentially carryovers from WWII rations made palatable for the consumer. Incidentally, it was also around then that I believe the term "mystery meat" was first invented.

In 1963, McDonald's began advertising meals for families. It was a milestone for marketing and public relations, as well as a paradigm shift—the idea that this type of fast food was appropriate for family dining, that you could get an inexpensive meal outside the home in a fast-food restaurant. Until then, people looked on fast food as inferior, but through this marketing coup, fast food became integral to the American diet. This meant more soda pop, more beef, more fries, and more saturated fat for the nation's consumers.

By 1965, canned soda pop was available in vending machines, and diet and regular soda came in many flavors. No longer just soda-fountain drinks, these beverages were available twenty-four hours a day, seven days a week, for anybody who had a dime and a nickel.

In 1966, the American Bottlers of Carbonated Beverages changed its name to the National Soft Drink Association and went on to become a powerful lobby, successfully fighting consumer groups that attempted to limit access to soda pop in venues such as public schools. In 2004, it changed its name again, this time to the American Beverage Association. In 2009, the ABA spent over $19 million on marketing, promotion, and lobbying, with twenty-five lobbyists at seven different firms on its payroll—an increase in spending of 1,000 percent over the previous election cycle.[141] Recently, they have helped defeat laws to raise taxes on high-sugar drinks. You can read more about this online at the Center for Responsive Politics—"Lobbying 2009: American Beverage Association."[141]

When high-fructose corn syrup (HFCS) was introduced in the late 1960s, our food supply really changed. Within two decades, it found its way into use in American soda products and other sweetened beverages, as well as other food products. HFCS is more fattening (more calories, ounce per ounce, than sugar) and less expensive than sugar. Since the introduction of HFCS, the public's consumption of it has grown to equal that of cane and beet sugar. It has recently become a target in America's battle against the obesity epidemic. Once HFCS became an ingredient in soda, soda became more fattening and higher in low-glycemic sugar.

In response to an outbreak of botulism in 1973, Congress passed Title 21, a law giving the Food and Drug Administration the power to regulate canned and bottled goods that crossed state lines.

The introduction of "New Coke" in 1985 was met with loud boos and great disdain by angry "Coke-aholics," who complained that it was a syrupy drink without any kick. Coke lovers called it "worse than Pepsi." At the time, I knew that the "new" Coke was simply a ruse to substitute high-fructose syrup for sugar. Indeed, when "Coke Classic" returned to the market and "New Coke" disappeared, corn syrup had been successfully substituted for real sugar, completing one of the most brilliant cost-savings ploys in manufacturing and marketing history.

In 1990, Congress passed the Nutrition Labeling and Information Act to help guide consumers in making healthy choices about the food they purchase, and to encourage manufacturers to produce healthier products. It suggests a dawning realization that consumers have a right to know what, exactly, they are eating.

By 2003, the obesity epidemic was national news, with a focus on saturated fat and low-glycemic sugar. Meanwhile, despite all the labeling efforts, Americans continued to consume a large portion of their calories from "junk food."

In 2009, the average annual sugar intake per person was a staggering 142 pounds, the average sodium intake per day was 4500 mg, and the average daily saturated fat intake was approximately 20 grams.[142]

## The FDA's "Good Manufacturing Practices"

Title 21 underwent major revisions and was expanded in 1979 with the creation of "Good Manufacturing Practices." These practices set higher levels of certain food additives and acidity levels in prepackaged food to discourage bacterial growth and reduce the likelihood of bacterial contamination. The idea that acidification of the food supply might have adverse consequences was not considered in any of the documented discussions about food safety.[143]

The acidification of food has long been used as a means to preserve it, but it wasn't until the modern era that the process evolved to prevent and regulate bacterial growth in food traveling long distances to sit on a store shelf. The FDA's system of "Good Manufacturing Practices" through Title 21 regulations does not regulate what acids and preservatives within a broad group are used; it only requires the pH to be below 4.6, a level low enough to discourage most bacteria. In fact, Title 21 *encourages* acidification of foods and beverages to pH 4.0 and below:

> *"Acidified foods shall be so manufactured, processed, and packaged that a finished equilibrium pH value of 4.6 or lower is achieved . . . If the finished equilibrium pH is 4.0 or below, then the measurement of acidity of the final product may be made by any suitable method."*
> [April 1, 2002; U.S. Government Printing Office, 21CFR114.80]

That sentence implies that the FDA is incentivizing manufacturers to acidify their product to pH <4.0. "Any suitable method" would presumably allow testing with just a pH meter to show that the pH was less than 4.0.

## Food and Drug Administration (FDA) Approved Food Additives

A corollary question to consider is what kind of food additives are being used to achieve these FDA-regulated acidity levels. It turns out there are 333 substances that are FDA approved—they are affectionately referred to as GRAS, for "Generally Recognized as Safe."[144, 145]

In February 2010, the Government Accountability Office[146] (GAO), a non-partisan group appointed by Congress to investigate federal agencies, published a scathing report to Congress.

Here is the first paragraph of "Food Safety: FDA Should Strengthen Its Oversight of Food Ingredients Determined to Be Generally Recognized as Safe (GRAS)."[147]

> *"FDA's oversight process does not help ensure the safety of all new GRAS ("Generally Recognized as Safe") determinations. FDA only reviews those GRAS determinations that companies submit to the agency's voluntary*

*notification program—the agency generally does not have information about other GRAS determinations companies have made because companies are not required to inform FDA of them. Furthermore, FDA has not taken certain steps that could help ensure the safety of GRAS determinations, particularly those about which the agency has not been notified. FDA has not issued guidance to companies on how to document their GRAS determinations or monitored companies to ensure that they have conducted GRAS determinations appropriately. Lastly, FDA has yet to issue a final regulation for its 1997 proposed rule that sets forth the framework and criteria for the voluntary notification program, potentially detracting from the program's credibility.*"

This states that not only was there inadequate oversight of the approval process, but that food manufacturers themselves and not the FDA were left to determine the "safety" of the additives they chose to employ in their products. For all intents and purposes, this process is industry self-regulated, providing the food additives comply with the list of approved GRAS substances. This is like asking tobacco manufacturers to tell us whether cigarette smoke is harmful or not.

Throughout the scientific community and in the literature and published reports dealing with food safety and food additives, we have not seen concerns raised about the possible adverse health consequences of food acidification. By the way, 13 percent of the GRAS substances are acids, including hydrochloric acid, which is considered a safe food additive.

An interesting report in September 2009 from the Ohio State Medical Center found that the age-adjusted incidence of all cancers among Amish adults in Ohio was 60 percent that of other adults, and only 37 percent of the control group for "tobacco-related" cancers[139]—including of the pharynx, larynx, and esophagus. In addition to the fact that the Amish drink and smoke less, the authors never specifically discussed the role of diet. We suggest that one possible explanation for the favorable cancer rates among the Amish is that they don't eat highly acidified and preservative-laden food.[139]

It is important to remember that reflux causes many different symptoms other than heartburn and indigestion. Silent reflux affects the voice box, throat, and lungs, and causes symptoms of cough, sore throat, hoarseness, and asthma, among others. Those are the most common symptoms for which people see doctors in America. Therefore, it is important for both doctors and patients to recognize that reflux is not always classic reflux (gastroesophageal disease, GERD). Based upon the author's experience, it is likely that reflux is grossly underdiagnosed and undertreated. For a review of the symptoms, see "How Do I Know if I Have Reflux?" on page 31.

## Summary and Conclusions

Why is reflux epidemic and why are esophageal cancer rates soaring? The cell biology (basic science) of reflux in conjunction with clinical experience has shown that a highly acidic diet is harmful for people with reflux. Amazing as it may seem, until now no one has investigated this problem, but even more amazingly no one has ever considered the possibility that there might be adverse health consequences of systemic acidification of America's food.

We believe that acidic food is indeed the reason reflux is epidemic and the reason that esophageal cancer (and pre-cancer, i.e., Barrett's esophagus) is increasing in prevalence so dramatically. From our point of view, we try to eat fresh, organic, nonprocessed foods and generally avoid acids. For most people, there is probably a middle road—having a glass of orange juice or soda pop once in a while doesn't cause reflux disease—but if that's all you drink day in and day out, it's likely to be a problem. For people with known reflux disease, a period of "acid/pepsin detox" makes good sense.

People will ask if we have proven these claims beyond a reasonable doubt —that dietary acid causes disease. We respond that we have cited here sound scientific evidence and the state of the art of clinical medicine. We believe that our data are compelling and speak for themselves. It is likely that we are dealing with an important public health issue. Yes, we are worried about the implications of all this, aren't you?

# References

1. Koufman JA. The Otolaryngologic manifestations of gastroesophageal reflux disease (GERD): A clinical investigation of 225 patients using ambulatory 24-hour pH monitoring and an experimental investigation of the role of acid and pepsin in the development of laryngeal injury. Laryngoscope 101 (Suppl. 53):1–78, 1991.
2. Koufman JA, Aviv JE, Casiano RR, Shaw GY. Laryngopharyngeal reflux: Position statement of the Committee on Speech, Voice and Swallowing Disorders of the American Academy of Otolaryngology—Head and Neck Surgery. Otolaryngol Head Neck Surg 127:32–35, 2002.
3. Koufman JA. Perspectives on laryngopharyngeal reflux: From silence to omnipresence. In *Classics in Voice and Laryngology*. Branski R, Sulica L, Eds. PP 179–189, Plural Publishing, San Diego, 2009.
4. Little FB, Koufman JA, Kohut RI, Marshal RB. Effect of gastric acid on the pathogenesis of subglottic stenosis. Ann of Otol Rhinol Laryngol 94:516–519, 1985.
5. Wiener GJ, Copper JB, Wu WC, Koufman JA, Richter JE, Castell DO. Is hoarseness an atypical manifestation of gastroesophogeal reflux? Gastroenterology 90:A1691, 1986.
6. Koufman JA, Wiener GJ, Wu WC, Castell DO. Reflux laryngitis and its sequelae: The diagnostic role of 24-hour pH monitoring. J Voice 2:78–89, 1988.
7. Weiner GJ, Koufman JA, Wu WC, *et al.* Chronic hoarseness secondary to gastroesophageal reflux disease: Documentation with 24-H ambulatory pH monitoring. Am J Gastroenterol 84:12, 1989.
8. Koufman JA. Aerodigestive manifestations of gastroesophageal reflux. What we don't yet know. Chest 104:1321-1322, 1993.
9. Koufman JA, Cummins MM. Reflux and early laryngeal carcinoma. Presented at the annual meeting of the Southern Section of the Triological Society. Key West, FL. January 6, 1995.
10. Koufman JA, Sataloff RT, Toohill R. Laryngopharyngeal reflux: Consensus report. J Voice 10:215–216, 1996.
11. Loughlin CJ, Koufman JA. Paroxysmal laryngospasm secondary to gastroesophageal reflux. Laryngoscope 106:1502–1505, 1996.
12. Loughlin CJ, Koufman JA, Averill DB, Cummins MM, Yong-Jae K, Little JP, Miller Jr. IJ, Meredith W. Acid-induced laryngospasm in a canine model. Laryngoscope 106:1506–1509, 1996.
13. Koufman JA. Methods and compositions for the diagnosis of extraesophageal reflux. United States Patent 5,879,897, 1996.
14. Koufman JA, Burke AJ. The etiology and pathogenesis of laryngeal carcinoma. Oto Clin N A 30:1–19, 1997.
15. Little JP, Matthews BL, Glock MS, Koufman JA, Reboussin DM, Loughlin CJ, McGuirt Jr. WF. Extraesophageal pediatric reflux: 24-hour double-probe pH monitoring of 222 children. Ann Otol Rhinol Laryngol Suppl 169: 1–16, 1997.

16. Matthews BL, Little JP, McGuirt Jr. WF, Koufman JA. Reflux in infants with laryngomalacia: Results of 24-hour double-probe pH monitoring. Otolaryngol Head Neck Surg 120:860–864, 1999.
17. Koufman JA, Amin M, Panetti M. Prevalence of reflux in 113 consecutive patients with laryngeal and voice disorders. Otolaryngol Head Neck Surg 123:385–388, 2000.
18. Reulbach TR, Belafsky PC, Blalock PD, Koufman JA, Postma GN. Occult laryngeal pathology in a community-based cohort. Otolaryngol Head Neck Surg 124:448–450, 2001.
19. Belafsky PC, Postma GN, Koufman JA. Laryngopharyngeal reflux symptoms improve before changes in physical findings. Laryngoscope 111: 979–981, 2001.
20. Belafsky PC, Postma GN, Koufman JA. The validity and reliability of the reflux finding score (RFS). Laryngoscope 111:1313–1317, 2001.
21. Amin MR, Koufman JA. Vagal neuropathy after upper respiratory infection: a viral etiology? Am J Otolaryngol 22:251–256, 2001.
22. Duke SG, Postma GN, McGuirt Jr. WF, Ririe D, Averill DB, Koufman JA. Laryngospasm and diaphragmatic arrest in the immature canine after laryngeal acid exposure: A possible model for sudden infant death syndrome (SIDS). Ann Otol Rhinol Laryngol 110:729–733, 2001.
23. Amin MR, Postma GN, Johnson P, Digges N, Koufman JA. Proton pump inhibitor resistance in the treatment of laryngopharyngeal reflux. Otolaryngol Head Neck Surg 125:374–378, 2001.
24. Belafsky PC, Postma GN, Daniels E, Koufman JA. Transnasal esophagoscopy. Otolaryngol Head Neck Surg 125:588–589, 2001.
25. Johnson PE, Koufman JA, Nowak LJ, Belafsky PC, Postma GN. Ambulatory 24-hour double-probe pH monitoring: The importance of manometry. Laryngoscope 111:1970–1975, 2001.
26. Smoak BR, Koufman JA. Effects of gum chewing on pharyngeal and esophageal pH. Ann Otol Rhinol Laryngol 110:1117–1119, 2001.
27. Postma GN, Tomek MS, Belafsky PC, Koufman JA. Esophageal motor function in laryngopharyngeal reflux is superior to that of classic gastroesophageal reflux disease. Ann Otol Rhinol Laryngol 110:1114–1116, 2001.
28. Axford SE, Sharp S, Ross PE, Pearson JP, Dettmar PW, Panetti M, Koufman JA. Cell biology of laryngeal epithelial defenses in health and disease: Preliminary studies. Ann Otol Rhinol Laryngol 110:1099–1108, 2001.
29. Belafsky PC, Postma GN, Koufman JA. Transnasal esophagoscopy (TNE). Otolaryngol Head Neck Surg 125: 588–589, 2001.
30. Belafsky PC, Postma GN, Koufman JA. Subglottic edema (pseudosulcus) as a manifestation of laryngopharyngeal reflux. Otolaryngol Head Neck Surg 126:649–652, 2002.
31. Belafsky PC, Postma GN, Koufman JA. Validity and reliability of the reflux symptom index (RSI). J Voice 16:274–277, 2002.

32. Koufman JA. Laryngopharyngeal reflux is different from classic gastroesophageal reflux disease. Ear Nose Throat J. 81:7–9 2002.

33. Koufman JA, Belafsky PC, Daniel E, Bach KK, Postma GN. Prevalence of esophagitis in patients with pH-documented laryngopharyngeal reflux. Laryngoscope 112:1606–1609, 2002.

34. Belafsky PC, Postma GN, Koufman JA. Hiatal hernia. Ear Nose Throat J. 81:502, 2002.

35. Koufman JA. Laryngopharyngeal reflux 2002: A new paradigm of airway disease. Ear Nose Throat J 81(9 Suppl 2) 2406, 2002.

36. Cohen JT, Bach KK, Postma GN, Koufman JA. Clinical manifestations of laryngopharyngeal reflux. Ear Nose Throat J. 81:14–23, 2002.

37. Postma GN, Johnson LF, Koufman JA. Treatment of laryngopharyngeal reflux. Ear Nose Throat J. 81:24–6, 2002.

38. Holland BW, Koufman JA, Postma GN, McGuirt Jr. WF. Laryngopharyngeal reflux and laryngeal web formation in patients with pediatric recurrent respiratory papillomas. Laryngoscope 112:1926–29, 2002.

39. Johnston N, Bulmer D, Gill GA, Panetti M, Ross PE, Pearson JP, Pignatelli M, Axford A, Dettmar PW, Koufman JA. Cell biology of laryngeal epithelial defenses in health and disease: Further studies. Ann Otol Rhinol Laryngol 112:481–491, 2003.

40. Cohen JT, Postma GN, Enriquez PS, Koufman JA. Barrett's Esophagus. Ear Nose Throat J. 82:422, 2003.

41. Westcott CJ, Hopkins MB, Bach KK, Postma GN, Belafsky PC, Koufman, JA. Fundoplication for laryngopharyngeal reflux. J American College of Surgeons 199: 23–30, 2004.

42. Johnston N, Knight J, Dettmar PW, Lively MO, Koufman J. Pepsin and carbonic anhydrase isoenzyme III as diagnostic markers for laryngopharyngeal reflux disease. Laryngoscope 114:2129–34, 2004.

43. Halum SL, Butler SG, Koufman JA, Postma GN. Treatment of globus by upper esophageal sphincter injection with botulinum toxin A. ENT J Ear Nose Throat J 84:74, 2005.

44. Postma GN, Cohen JT, Belafsky PC, Halum SL, Gupta SK, Bach KK, Koufman JA. Transnasal esophagoscopy revisited (over 700 consecutive cases). Laryngoscope 115:321–3, 2005.

45. Carrau RL, Khidr A, Gold KF, Crawley JA, Hillson EM, Koufman JA, Pashos CL. Validation of a quality-of-life instrument for laryngopharyngeal reflux. Arch Otolaryngol Head Neck Surg 131:315–20, 2005.

46. Halum SL, Postma GN, Johnston C, Belafsky PC, Koufman JA. Patients with isolated laryngopharyngeal reflux are not obese. Laryngoscope 115:1042–5, 2005.

47. Knight J, Lively MO, Johnston N, Dettmar PW, Koufman JA. Sensitive pepsin immunoassay for detection of laryngopharyngeal reflux. Laryngoscope 115:1473–8, 2005.

48. Johnston N, Dettmar PW, Lively MO, Postma GN, Belafsky PC, Birchall M, Koufman JA. Effect of pepsin on laryngeal stress protein (Sep70, Sep53, and Hsp70) response: Role in laryngopharyngeal reflux disease. Ann Otol Rhinol Laryngol 115:47–58, 2005.

49. Gill GA, Johnston N, Buda A, Pignatelli M, Pearson J, Dettmar PW, Koufman JA. Laryngeal epithelial defenses against laryngopharyngeal reflux (LPR): Investigations of pepsin, carbonic anhydrase III, pepsin, and the inflammatory response. Ann Otol Rhinol Laryngol 114:913–21, 2005.
50. Koufman JA, Johnston WC, Wright SC. Laryngopharyngeal reflux is worse in smokers than non-smokers. (Unreported data 2005).
51. Johnston N, Dettmar PW, Lively MO, Koufman JA. Effect of pepsin on laryngeal stress protein (Sep70, Sep53, and Hsp70) response: Role in laryngopharyngeal reflux disease. Ann Otol Rhinol Laryngol 115:47–58, 2006.
52. Halum SL, Postma GN, Bates DD, Koufman JA. Incongruence between histologic and endoscopic diagnoses of Barrett's Esophagus using transnasal esophagoscopy. Laryngoscope. 116:303–6, 2006.
53. Johnston N, Dettmar PW, Lively MO, Koufman JA. Effect of pepsin on laryngeal stress protein (Sep70, Sep53, and Hsp70) response: Role in laryngopharyngeal reflux disease. Ann Otol Rhinol Laryngol. 115:47–58, 2006.
54. Johnston N, Dettmar PW, Bishwokarma B, Lively MO, Koufman JA. Activity/stability of human pepsin: Implications for reflux attributed laryngeal disease. Laryngoscope. 117:1036–9, 2007.
55. Koufman JA, Lively MO, Rubin M, Nelson D, Johnston N, Bishwokarma B, Wright SC. Use of a sensitive ELISA for the detection of pepsin in the airway secretions of patients with laryngopharyngeal reflux (LPR), gastroesophageal reflux disease (GERD), and healthy controls. Presented at the Annual Meeting of the American Broncho-Esophagological Association. Orlando, FL. May 2, 2008.
56. Rees LE, Pazmany L, Gutowska-Owsiak D, Inman CF, Phillips A, Stokes CR, Johnston N, Koufman JA, Postma G, Bailey M, Birchall MA. The mucosal immune response to laryngopharyngeal reflux. Am J Respir Crit Care Med. 177:1187–93, 2008.
57. Birchall MA, Bailey M, Gutowska-Owsiak D, Johnston N, Inman CF, Stokes CR, Postma G, Pazmary L, Koufman JA, Phillips A, Rees LE. Immunologic response of the laryngeal mucosa to extraesophageal reflux. Ann Otol Rhinol Laryngol 117:891–5, 2008.
58. Amin MR, Postma GN, Setzen M, Koufman JA. Transnasal esophagoscopy: A position statement from the American Bronchoesophagological Association (ABEA). Otolaryngol Head Neck Surg 138:411–13, 2008.
59. Koufman JA, Block C. Differential diagnosis of paradoxical vocal fold movement. American Journal of Speech and Hearing 17:327–34, 2008.
60. Winkelstein A. Peptic esophagitis: A new clinical entity. JAMA 104:906-909, 1935.
61. Allison PR. Reflux esophogitis, sliding hiatal hernia, and the anatomy of repair. Surg Gynecol Obstet 1951: 92:419–431.
62. Nissen R. Gastopexy and "fundoplication" in surgical treatment of hiatal hernia. Am J Dig Dis 6:954–961, 1961.
63. Hunter J. Laparoscopic fundoplication. Ann Surg 223:673–687, 1996.
64. Fyke FE, Code CF, Schlegel JF. The gastroesophageal sphincter in healthy human beings. Gastroenterologia [Basel] 86:135–150, 1956.

65. Gerhardt DC, Shuck TJ, Bordeaux RA, Winship DH. Human upper esophageal sphincter. Response to volume, osmotic and acid stimuli. Gastroenterology 75:268–274, 1978.
66. Burnett W. An evaluation of the gastroduodenal fibrescope. Gut 3:361–365, 1962.
67. Miller FA, Dovale J, Gunther T. Utilization of inlying pH probe for evaluation of acid-peptic diathesis. Arch Surg 89:199–203, 1964.
68. Spencer, J. Prolonged pH recording in the study of gastroesophageal reflux. Br J Surg, 56:912–914, 1969.
69. DeMeester TR, Johnson LF, Joseph GJ, Toscano MS, Hall AW, Skinner DB. Patterns of gastroesophageal reflux in health and disease. Ann Surg 184: 459–470, 1976.
70. Helm JF, Dodds WJ, Riedel DR, *et al.* Determinants of esophageal acid clearance in normal subjects. Gastroenterol 85:607–12, 1983.
71. Rogers E, Goldkind S, Isri O, *et al.* Adenocarcinoma of the lower esophagus. A disease primarily of white men with Barrett's Esophagus. J Clin Gastroenterol 8:613–618 1986.
72. Vitale GC, Cheadle WG, Patel B, *et al.* The effect of alcohol on nocturnal gastroesophageal reflux. JAMA 258:2077–2079, 1987.
73. Klinkenberg-Knol EC, Meuwissen SG. Treatment of reflux oesophagitis resistant to H2-receptor antagonists. Digestion (Supplement 1):47–53, 1989.
74. Korsten MA, Rosman AS, Fishbein S, *et al.* Chronic xerostomia increases esophageal acid exposure and is associated with esophageal injury. Am J Med 90:701–706, 1990.
75. Peghini PL, Katz PO, Bracy NA, Castell DO. Nocturnal recovery of gastric acid secretion with twice daily dosing of proton pump inhibitors. Am J Gastroenterol 93:763–767, 1998.
76. Korsten MA, Rosman AS, Fishbein S, Shlein RD, Goldberg HE, Biener A. Chronic xerostomia increases esophageal acid exposure and is associated with esophageal injury. Am J Med. 90:701–706, 1991.
77. Chiverton SG, Howden CW, Burget DW, Hunt RH. Omeprazole (20 mg) daily given in the morning or evening: A comparison of effects on gastric acidity, and plasma gastrin and omeprazole concentration. Aliment Pharmacol Ther. 6:103–111, 1992.
78. Jones AT, Balan KK, Jenkins SA, *et al.* Assay of gastricsin and individual pepsins in human gastric juice. J Clin Pathol. 46:254–258, 1993.
79. Leite LP, Johnston BT, Just RJ, Castell DO. Persistent acid secretion during omeprazole therapy: A study of gastric acid profiles in patients demonstrating failure of omeprazole therapy. Am J Gastroenterol 91:1527–1531, 1996.
80. Ho KY, Kang JY, Seow A. Prevalence of gastrointestinal symptoms in a multiracial Asian population, with particular reference to reflux-type symptoms. Am J Gastroenterol 93:1816–1822, 1998.
81. Peghini PL, Katz PO, Bracy NA, Castell DO. Nocturnal recovery of gastric acid secretion with twice daily dosing of proton pump inhibitors. Am J Gastroenterol. 93:763–767, 1998.
82. Maton PN, Orlando R, Joelsson B. Efficacy of omeprazole versus ranitidine for symptomatic treatment of poorly responsive acid reflux disease—a prospective, controlled trial. Aliment Pharmacol Ther. 13:819–826, 1999.

83. Jansen JB, Van Oene JC. Standard-dose lansoprazole is more effective than high-dose ranitidine in achieving endoscopic healing and symptom relief in patients with moderately severe reflux oesophagitis. The Dutch Lansoprazole Study Group. Aliment Pharmacol Ther. 13:1611–1620, 1999.
84. El-Serag HB, Petersen NJ, Carter J, *et al.* Gastroesophageal reflux among different racial groups in thc Unitcd States. Gastroenterology 126:1692–1699, 2004.
85. Tambankar AP, Peters JH, Portale G, Hsieb C-C, Hagen JA, Bremner CG, DeMeester TR. Omeprazole does not reduce gastroesophageal reflux: New insights using multichannel impedance technology. J Gastroenterol Surg 8: 888–895, 2004.
86. Kawamura O, Aslam M, Rittmann T, *et al.* Physical and pH properties of gastroesophagopharyngeal refluxate: A 24-hour simultaneous ambulatory impedance and pH monitoring study. Am J Gastroenterol. 99:1000–10, 2004.
87. Lam P, Wei WI, Hui Y, Ho WK. Prevalence of pH-documented laryngopharyneal reflux in Chinese patients with clinically suspected reflux laryngitis. Am J Otolaryngol 27: 186–9, 2006.
88. Jackson, C. *The Life of Chevalier Jackson: An Autobiography.* Macmillan Co., New York, p. 229, 1938.
89. Aviv JE, Takoudes TG, Ma G, *et al.* Office-based esophagoscopy: A preliminary report. Otolaryngol Head Neck Surg 125:170–5, 2001.
90. Jobe BA, Hunter JG, Chang EY, *et al.* Office-based unsedated small caliber endoscopy is equivalent to conventional sedated endoscopy in screening and surveillance for Barrett's Esophagus: A randomized and blinded comparison. Am J Gastroenterol 101:2693703, 2006.
91. Cherry J, Margulies SI. Contact ulcer of the larynx. Laryngoscope 78:1937–1940, 1968.
92. Delahunty JE, Ardan G. Globus hystericus—a manifestation of reflux oesophagitis? J Laryngol Otol 84:1049–1054, 1970.
93. Delahunty JE. Acid laryngitis. J Laryngol Otol 86:335–342, 1972.
94. Chodosh PL. Gastro-esophago-pharyngeal reflux. Laryngoscope 87:1418–1427, 1977.
95. Fearon B, Bram I. Esophageal hiatal hernia in infants and children. Ann Otol Rhinol Laryngol 90: 387–391, 1981.
96. Olson NR. Effects of stomach acid on the larynx. Proc Am Laryngol Assoc 104:108–112, 1983.
97. Bain WM, Harrington JW, Thomas LE, Schaefer SD. Head and neck manifestations of gastroesophageal reflux. Laryngoscope 1983: 93:175–9.
98. Ossakow SJ, Elta G, Colturi T, Bogdasarian R, Nostrant TT. Esophageal reflux and dysmotility as the basis for persistent cervical symptoms. Ann Otol Rhinol Laryngol 96:387–392, 1987.
99. Gaynor EB. Gastroesophageal reflux as an etiologic factor in laryngeal complications of intubation. Laryngoscope 98:972–979, 1988.
100. Ward PH, Berci G. Observations on the pathogenesis of chronic non-specific pharyngitis and laryngitis. Laryngoscope 92:1377–1382, 1988.
101. Toohill RJ, Kuhn JC. Role of refluxed acid in pathogenesis of laryngeal disorders. Am J Med 103:100S–106S, 1997.

102. Kuhn J, Toohill RJ, Ulualp SO, *et al.* Pharyngeal acid reflux events in patients with vocal cord nodules. Laryngoscope 108:1146–1149, 1998.

103. DelGaudio JM. Direct nasopharyngeal reflux of gastric acid is a contributing factor in refractory chronic rhinosinusitis. Laryngoscope 115:946–57, 2005.

104. Gaynor EB. Gastroesophageal reflux as an etiologic factor in laryngeal complications of intubation. Laryngoscope 98:972–979, 1988.

105. Smit CF, Mathus-Vliegen LM, Devriese PP, *et al.* Monitoring of laryngopharyngeal reflux: influence of meals and beverages. Ann Otol Rhinol Laryngol 112: 109–12, 2003.

106. Eryuksel E, Dogan M, Golabi P, Sehitoglu MA, Celikel T. Treatment of laryngopharyngeal reflux improves asthma symptoms in asthmatics. J Asthma 43:539–42, 2006.

107. Sweet MP, Patti MG, Leard LE, Golden JA, Hays SR, Hoopes C, Theodore PR. Gastroesophageal reflux in patients with idiopathic pulmonary fibrosis referred for lung transplantation. J Thorac Cardiovasc Surg 133: 1078–84, 2007.

108. Wetmore RF. Effects of acid on the larynx of the maturing rabbit and their possible significance to the sudden infant death syndrome. Laryngoscope 103:1242–54, 1993.

109. Ross JA, Noordzji JP, Woo P. Voice disorders in patients with suspected laryngopharyngeal reflux disease. J Voice 12:84–88, 1998.

110. Rothstein SG. Reflux and vocal disorders in singers with bulemia. J Voice 12:89–90, 1998.

111. Grontved AM, West F. pH monitoring in patients with benign voice disorders. Acta Otolaryngol Suppl 543:229–231, 2000.

112. Noordzij JP, Khidr A, Desper E, *et al.* Correlation of pH probe-measured laryngopharyngeal reflux with symptoms and signs of reflux laryngitis. Laryngoscope 112: 2192–5, 2002.

113. Tokashiki R, Nakamura K, Watanabe Y, Yamaguchi H, Suzuki M. The relationship between esophagoscopic findings and total acid reflux time below pH 4 and pH 5 in the upper esophagus in patients with laryngopharyngeal reflux disease (LPRD). Auris Nasus Larynx 32:265–8, 2005.

114. Garcia I, Krishna P, Rosen CA. Severe laryngeal hyperkeratsosis secondary to laryngopharyngeal reflux. Ear Nose Throat J 85:417, 2006.

115. Park KH, Choi SM, Kwon SU, *et al.* Diagnosis of laryngopharyngeal reflux among globus patients. Otolaryngol Head Neck Surg 134: 81–5, 2006.

116. Payne RJ, Kost KM, Frenkiel S, Zeitouni AG, *et al.* Laryngeal inflammation assessed using the reflux finding score in obstructive sleep apnea. Otolaryngol Head Neck Surg 134: 836–42, 2006.

117. Fenton JE, Kieran SM. Re: Nasopharyngitis is a clinical sign of laryngopharyngeal reflux. Am J Rhinol 21:135, 2007.

118. Tsunoda K, Ishimoto S, Suzuki M, *et al.* An effective management regimen for laryngeal granuloma caused by gastro-esophageal reflux: Combination therapy with suggestions for lifestyle modifications. Acta Otolaryngol 127:88–92, 2007.

119. Ward PH, Hanson DG. Reflux as an etiological factor of carcinoma of the laryngopharynx. Laryngoscope 98:1195–1199, 1988.

120. Morrison MD. Is chronic gastroesophageal reflux a causative factor in glottic carcinoma? Otolaryngol Head Neck Surg 99:370–373, 1988.

121. Geterud A, Bove M, Ruth M. Hypopharyngeal acid exposure: An independent risk factor for laryngeal cancer? Laryngoscope 113:2201–5, 2003.

122. Dagli S, Dagli U, Kurtaran H, Alkim C, Sahin B. Laryngopharyngeal reflux in laryngeal cancer. Turk J Gastroenterol 15:77–81, 2004.

123. Ozlugedik S, Yorulmaz I, Gokcan K. Is laryngopharyngeal reflux an important risk factor in the development of laryngeal carcinoma? Eur Arch Otorhinolaryngol 263:339–43, 2006.

124. Johnston N, Yan J, Samuels TL. Pepsin, at pH7 in non-acidic laryngopharyngeal refluxate, significantly alters the expression of multiple genes implicated in carcinogensis. Presented at the annual meeting of the American Broncho-Esophogological Association, Las Vegas NV, April 28, 2010. (Submitted for publication to The Annals of Otology, Rhinology and Laryngology.)

125. Piper DW, Fenton BH. pH stability and activity curves of pepsin with special reference to their clinical importance. Gut 6:506–508, 1965.

126. Goldberg HI, Dodds WJ, Gee S, *et al.* Role of acid and pepsin in acute experimental esophagitis. Gastroenterology 56:223–230, 1969.

127. Lillemoe KD, Johnson LF, Harmon JW. Role of the components of the gastroduodenal contents in experimental acid esophagitis. Surgery 92:276:–284, 1982.

128. Johnson LF, Harmon JW. Experimental esophagitis in a rabbit model. Clinical Relevance. J Clin Gastroenterol 8 (Suppl 1):26–44, 1986.

129. Samuels TL, Johnston N. Pepsin as a marker of extraesophageal reflux. Ann Otol Rhinol Laryngol 119:203–8, 2010.

130. Barrett NR. The lower esophagus lined by columnar epithelium. Surgery 41:881–894, 1957.

131. Conio M, Blanchi S, Lapertosa G, *et al.* Long-term endoscopic surveillance of patients with Barrett's Esophagus. Incidence of dysplasia and adenocarcinoma: A prospective study. Am J Gastroenterol 98:1931–9, 2003.

132. Rogers E, Goldkind S, Isri O, *et al.* Adenocarcinoma of the lower esophagus. A disease primarily of white men with Barrett's Esophagus. J Clin Gastroenterol 8:613–618, 1986.

133. Lagergren J, Bergstrom R, Lindgren A, Nyren O. Symptomatic gastroesophageal reflux as a risk factor for esophageal adenocarcinoma. NEJM. 340:825–831, 1999.

134. Reavis KM, Morris CD, Gopal DV, Hunter JG, Jobe BA. Laryngopharyngeal reflux symptoms better predict the presence of esophageal adenocarcinoma than typical gastroesophageal reflux symptoms. Ann Surg 239:849–56, 2004.

135. Wong A, Fitzgerald RC. Epidemiologic risk factors for Barrett's Esophagus and associated adenocarcinoma. Clin Gastroenterol Hepatology 3:1–10, 2005.

136. Koufman JA. Low-Acid Diet for Recalcitrant Laryngopharyngeal Reflux: Therapeutic Benefits and Their Implications. Ann Otol Rhinol Laryngol 120:281–87, 2011.
137. Koufman JA. The changing pattern of reflux in America: Disease prevalence is increasing and the typical laryngopharyngeal reflux (LPR) patient is getting younger. (Unreported data 2010).
138. Stanciu C, Bennett JR. Smoking and gastroesophageal reflux. Br Med J 3:793–95, 1972.
139. Westman JA, Ferketich A, Kauffman R, *et al.* Low cancer incidence rates in Ohio Amish. Cancer Causes Controls 211: 69–75, 2010.
140. Bellis M. Introduction to pop: The history of soft drinks timeline. About.com (http://inventors.about.com/od/sstartinventions/a/soft_drink.htm)
141. Lobbying 2009: American Beverage Association. Center for Responsive Politics. (http://www.opensecrets.org/lobby/clientlbs.php?year=2009&lname=American+Beverage+Assn&id) March, 2010.
142. United States Average Annual Sugar Intake. USDA Economic Research Service.(http://www.ers.usda.gov/Data/FoodConsumption/app/availability.aspx) January, 2008.
143. "Acidified Foods." Code of Federal Regulations—Title 21—Food and Drugs Chapter I, Department Of Health And Human Services Subchapter B—Food for Human Consumption Part 114. United States Food and Drug Administration. Arlington, VA, Washington Business Information, 2010.
144. Food and Drug Administration. Guidance for Industry: Frequently Asked Questions About GRAS (Generally Regarded as Safe) Food Additives. (http://www.fda.gov/Food/GuidanceComplianceRegulatoryInformation/GuidanceDocuments/FoodIngredientsandPackaging/ucm061846.htm)
145. "Generally Recognized as Safe Food Additives: FDA Database of Selected GRAS Substances." United States Food and Drug Administration. National Technical Information Service, Springfield, VA, 2009.
146. Walker D. GAO Answers the Question: What's in a Name? *United States Government Accountability Office. (http://www.gao.gov/about/rollcall07192004.pdf/) July, 2004.*
147. "Food Safety: FDA Should Strengthen Its Oversight of Food Ingredients Determined to Be Generally Recognized as Safe (GRAS)." GAO-10–246: United States Government Accountability Office, February 3, 2010.

# Acidity (pH) of Common Foods and Beverages

We tested the pH (acidity) of many foods and beverages. A pH of 7 is neutral (nonacidic), and pH 1 is very acidic. Stomach acid itself is usually between pH 1 and pH 4. For **The Reflux Diet,** foods and beverages below pH 4 are too acidic. In fact, for the two-week start-up induction period, we recommend avoiding anything with pH 5 or less. Remember, low pH means high acidity. Good pH values for foods and beverages you eat often should be pH 5–7. After induction, pH 4–5 foods are okay in moderation.

Please understand that we could not test every food and beverage on the market. You may find more information on the pH of some common foods, such as yogurts and dried fruits, on our website at www.refluxcookbookblog.com.

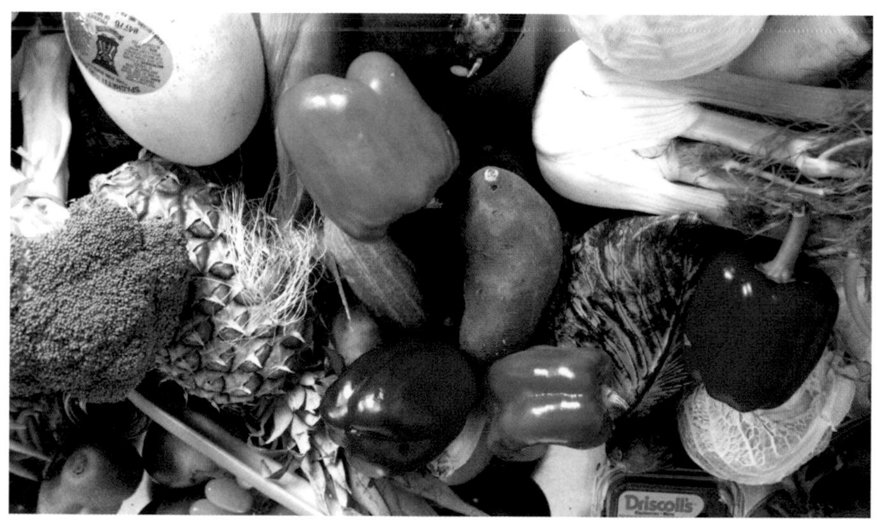

## SUMMARY TABLE:

### Red Is Bad & Green Is Good

(B means "Bad for Reflux" for reasons other than acidity)

| | pH |
|---|---|
| Agave nectar (Sweet Cactus Farms) | 4.5 |
| Apples – Fuji | 4.0 |
| Apples – Gala | 4.2 |
| Apples – Granny Smith | 3.6 |
| Apples – McIntosh | 3.7 |
| Apples – Macoun | 3.2 |
| Apples – Red Delicious | 4.2 |
| Applesauce (Mott's original) | 3.4 |
| Avocado | 7.8 |
| Banana | 5.6 |
| Barbecue sauce (Bull's-Eye original) | 3.7 |
| Barbecue sauce (Kraft original) | 3.4 |
| Beets – red | 6.1 |
| Bell pepper – green | 5.1 |
| Bell pepper – Italian stuffing pepper | 5.0 |
| Bell pepper – orange | 4.8 |
| Bell pepper – red | 4.9 |
| Blackberries | 3.7 |
| Blueberries | 3.7 |
| Bottled water (Poland Spring) | 6.9 |
| Broccoli – cooked | 6.2 |
| Broccoli – raw | 6.3 |
| Budweiser beer [B] | 4.5 |
| Cabbage – green | 6.0 |
| Cabbage – red | 6.3 |
| Cabbage – Savoy | 6.1 |
| Caesar dressing (Newman's Own) | 3.5 |
| Carrots | 7.0 |
| Cherries | 3.9 |
| Coca-Cola | 2.8 |
| Coca-Cola – diet | 3.7 |
| Pomegranate cranberry juice (Langer's) | 2.8 |
| Coffee (strong black) Limit one cup a day | 5.0 |
| Coffee (with milk) Limit one cup a day | 6.2 |
| Cognac | 3.0 |

| | |
|---|---|
| Coke Zero | 3.3 |
| Corn | 6.9 |
| Corn – whole kernel (Del Monte) | 6.6 |
| Cranberry juice (Tropicana) | 2.9 |
| Cranberry pomegranate juice (Knudsen) | 3.7 |
| Cream soda[B] (Dr. Brown's diet) | 4.5 |
| Cucumber | 6.0 |
| Diced tomatoes[B] (San Marzano) | 4.0 |
| Eggplant | 6.0 |
| Endive | 6.0 |
| Fennel | 6.9 |
| Gatorade (fruit punch) | 3.0 |
| Gherkin | 5.4 |
| Ginger | 6.5 |
| Grape – green, seedless | 3.6 |
| Grapefruit – pink | 3.4 |
| Green beans – canned, cut (Green Giant) | 5.2 |
| Green beans – cooked | 6.3 |
| Green beans – raw | 6.2 |
| Hot sauce (Texas Pete) | 3.1 |
| Iced tea (Lipton lemon) | 3.2 |
| Italian dressing (Zesty Kraft) | 5.2 |
| Ketchup (Heinz) | 3.4 |
| Kiwi | 3.4 |
| Lemon | 2.9 |
| Lime | 2.7 |
| Mandarin oranges (Dole) | 3.2 |
| Mango (Del Monte "Sunfresh mango in light syrup") | 3.4 |
| Mango | 3.7 |
| Melon – ripe cantaloupe | 6.1 |
| Milk – 2% organic | 7.5 |
| Milk – Lactaid fat-free | 7.0 |
| Milk[B] – whole, processed | 6.5 |
| Mountain Dew – diet | 3.1 |
| Mushrooms – domestic | 6.1 |
| Mushrooms – portobello | 6.5 |
| Mustard – Dijon (Grey Poupon) | 3.6 |
| Mustard – yellow (White Rose) | 3.2 |
| Nectarines | 3.3 |
| New York City tap water | 7.0 |
| Oatmeal with 2% milk | 7.2 |

| | |
|---|---|
| Olives – black, pitted (Best Brand) | 7.3 |
| Onion[B] – white | 6.0 |
| Onion[B] – Spanish yellow raw | 6.3 |
| Onion[B] – white sautéed | 6.4 |
| Orange – navel | 3.8 |
| Orange juice | 3.8 |
| Pancake batter – banana/oatmeal | 6.8 |
| Parsley – Italian flat leaf | 6.1 |
| Parsnip | 6.6 |
| Peaches | 3.6 |
| Pear – Bosc | 5.3 |
| Peas – canned, small (Le Sueur) | 5.8 |
| Pellegrino[B] | 4.8 |
| Pepsi | 3.5 |
| Pepsi – diet | 2.9 |
| Pickle – crunchy, dill (B&G) | 3.7 |
| Pineapple | 3.4 |
| Pomegranate | 3.3 |
| Potato – Idaho | 5.7 |
| Potato – Yukon gold | 6.0 |
| Prosecco (Mionetto) | 3.1 |
| Radish – red or black | 6.1 |
| Ranch dressing – reduced fat (Kraft) | 3.9 |
| Raspberries | 4.2 |
| Red Bull – energy drink | 3.9 |
| Russian dressing (Wishbone) | 3.8 |
| Salsa – mild chunky (Tostitos) | 3.7 |
| Salsa[B] – tomato chipotle (Rosa Mexicano) | 4.1 |
| Seltzer (Seagram's original) | 3.8 |
| Snapple – diet lemon | 3.3 |
| Sparkling water[B] (Poland Spring) | 4.3 |
| Sprite Zero – diet soda | 3.6 |
| Squash – acorn | 5.9 |
| Squash – spaghetti | 6.2 |
| Stolichnaya vodka[B] on the rocks (lemon twist) | 4.4 |
| Strawberries | 3.5 |
| Tab – diet soda | 2.9 |
| Tea (Chinese white jasmine) Limit one cup a day, mild brew | 5.6 |
| Thousand Island dressing (Kraft) | 3.6 |
| Tomato juice (Campbell's from concentrate) | 3.9 |
| Tomato paste[B] (Hunt) | 4.0 |

| | |
|---|---|
| Tomato sauce (Del Monte) | 3.9 |
| Tomato sauce[B] – mushroom (Prego Italian) | 4.0 |
| Tomato sauce[B] – organic (Del Monte) | 4.1 |
| Tomato sauce[B] – pizza quick (Ragú) | 4.1 |
| Tomatoes[B] – beefsteak cooked | 4.5 |
| Tomatoes[B] – Mexican cooked | 4.8 |
| Tomatoes[B] – Mexican | 4.3 |
| Tomatoes[B] – Roma (raw or cooked) | 4.4 |
| Tomatoes[B] – whole peeled (Best Yet) | 4.1 |
| Tomatoes – whole peeled (San Marzano) | 3.9 |
| Turnip | 6.2 |
| V8[B] vegetable juice | 4.2 |
| Vodka[B] (Absolut) | 4.7 |
| Worcestershire Sauce (Lea & Perrins) | 3.4 |
| Yams | 6.1 |
| Yogurt – 1% milk fat plain (Cream-O-Land) | 4.3 |
| Yogurt – 1% peach | 4.0 |
| Yogurt – peach, fruit on bottom (Dannon) Limit | 4.1 |
| Zucchini | 6.6 |

# About the Authors

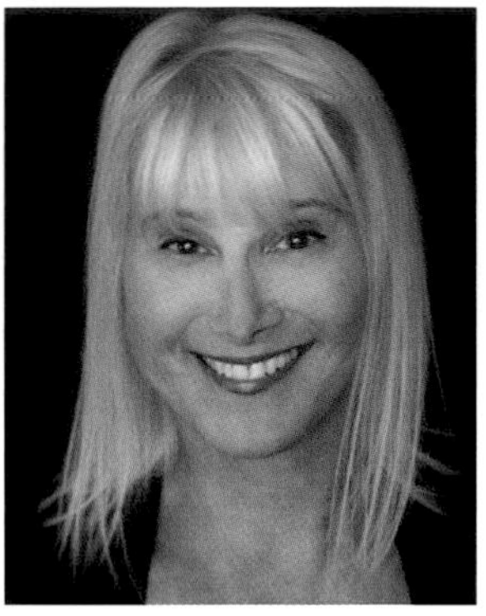

**Dr. Jamie Koufman** is one of the world's leading authorities on reflux and has lectured widely on the subject both nationally and internationally. For nearly three decades, her pioneering research has focused on reflux as it affects the voice and breathing passages. She coined the terms "silent reflux" and "laryngopharyngeal reflux (LPR)," the medical term for reflux that involves the larynx (voice box) and throat.

Dr. Koufman is the founder and director of the Voice Institute of New York, one of the premier comprehensive voice treatment centers in the United States. She is Professor of Clinical Otolaryngology at New York Medical College, and has been listed in Top Doctors in America every year since 1994. Dr. Koufman writes a medical blog on voice disorders, vocal cord surgery, reflux, and transnasal endoscopy; see www.VoiceInstituteofNewYork.com.

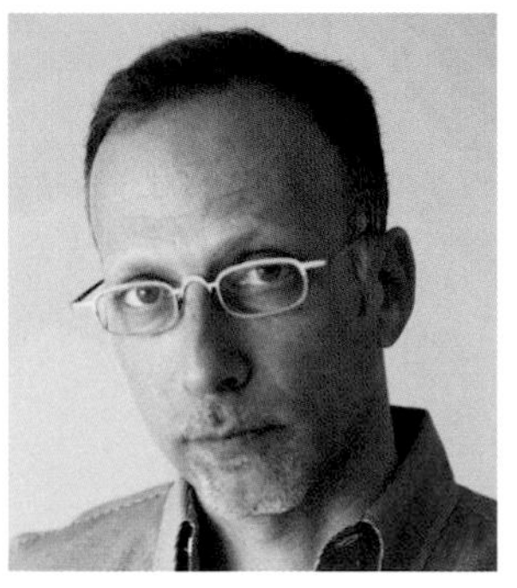

**Dr. Jordan Stern** is a board-certified otolaryngologist (head and neck surgeon) with over twenty years of experience in the management of upper airway diseases. He is also the founder and director of BlueSleep, a comprehensive sleep apnea and snoring center, and has assembled a multidisciplinary team dedicated to the treatment of sleep apnea and snoring in adults and children.

Dr. Stern has published and lectured widely on the subject of sleep apnea and head and neck tumors. He is past director of the Saint Vincent's Head and Neck Oncologic Surgery program and the New York Eye & Ear Infirmary's Head and Neck Surgery service. He has been featured in *The New York Times* "Top Docs" every year since 2007. Recently, he produced *Music for Dreams* with pianist Magdalena Baczewska (see www.bluesleep.com).

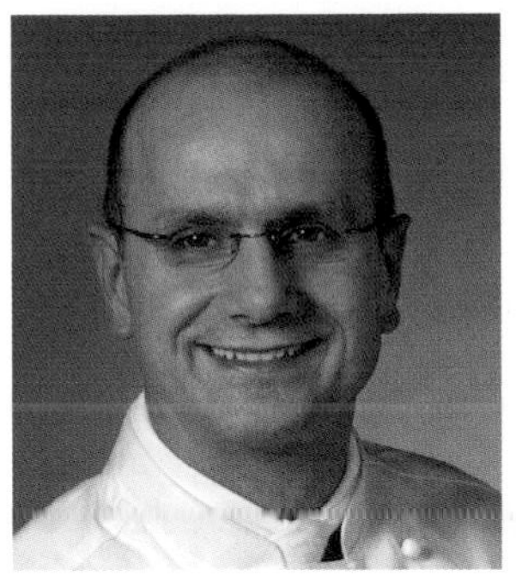

**Chef Marc Michel Bauer** is the Master Chef and Roundsman at the French Culinary Institute, where he has spent the past eighteen years honing his culinary and technical skills and engaging in his passion to educate and inspire. As a French Master Chef, he was formerly an executive chef at Délices de France in Manhattan. He earned a double Advanced Certification in Culinary Arts and Science in France, and a Bachelor of Science from SUNY College in New York.

Chef Bauer brings a wealth of creativity to cooking through his use of local ingredients and techniques acquired from his travels abroad, as well as his ability to design new dishes by adapting recipes to meet special dietary needs. He has worked side by side in his career with many of the industry's top chefs, including Alain Sailhac, Jacques Pépin, André Soltner, and Jacques Torres. Having experienced acid reflux personally, he recognized the need to create simple recipes that would enable people with reflux to enjoy their food and not be limited by dietary restrictions.

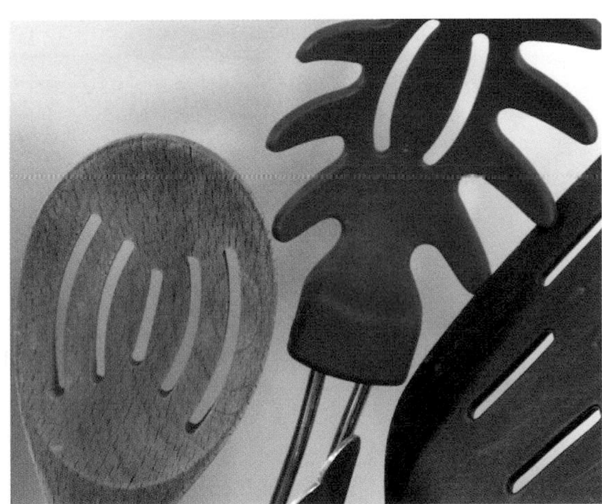

# Acknowledgments

The authors would like to recognize and thank some of the people who were instrumental in making this book successful: Greg VanHorn for research assistance: Jamie Bernard, Annabelle Day, and M. George Stevenson for editing; Tara Miller and Elpiniki Athanasiadou for calculating the nutritional values; and Ana Rogers and Gene Seidman for book design. Special thanks also to Mark Ballard, Latasha Taylor, Lana Baker, Julia Mankin, Sarah Hausman, and Meryl Moss.

# Index

Acid-free induction, 27, 28, 40, 45–47, 61, 166, 187
Acid reflux
  definitions, 11–13, 159–160
  history of reflux, 160–162
Acidification of food, 23–24, 173–176
Aerodigestive tract, 159
  specialty, 166–167
Agave nectar, 64, 155, 188
Alcohol, 28, 38, 47, 55, 56
  and sleep, 34
Aloe vera, 46, 50
  recipes
    Gala apple honeydew smoothie, 72
    No-alarm Mexican salsa, 134
    Tropical ginger and aloe rice pudding, 150
American Beverage Association (ABA), 171–173
American Bottlers of Carbonated Beverages (ABCB), 171
Amish, 175
Anti-reflux diet, 17, 65
Artificial sweeteners, 46
Asparagus, 52
  how to boil and shock, 97
  how to peel and dice, 94
  recipes
    Vegetarian sweet potato and lentil salad, 94
    Prosciutto-wrapped asparagus crêpes, 96
    Marc's kick-ass risotto with asparagus and morels, 115
    Asian pork stir-fry, 127
Atypical reflux disease, 13, 160

Bad reflux foods, 55–59
  pH table, 57, 188–191
Banana, 16, 45, 63
  pH, 188
  recipes
    Banana ginger energy smoothie, 71
    Breakfast couscous with fruit and poppy seeds, 73
    OMG banana oatmeal pancakes, 74
    Muesli-style oatmeal, 85
    No-alarm Mexican salsa, 134
    Awesome oatmeal cookies, 141
    Banana pumpkin tart, 145
    Banana with dates in filo dough, 146
    Honey, date, melon, banana, and basil crepe, 148
    Ginger crêpes with bananas and cantaloupe, 149
    Quick banana sorbet, 153
    Butterscotch praline mousse, 154
    Sweet potato and cantaloupe cake, 155
Barium swallow, 161, 162
Barrett's Esophagus, 40, 164, 166–170, 176
Beans, 52, 63, 64, 189
  recipes
    Crunchy cucumber and lentil salad, 90
    Sweet potato and green bean salad, 91
    Black bean and cilantro soup, 103
    Slow black bean soup, 103
    Scallops with penne verde, 112
    Medley of mussels, prosciutto, and fennel on whole-wheat pasta, 114
    One-pot vegetable and rice tofu, 116–117
    Chicken cutlet with prosciutto, 122
    Chicken south-of-the-border style, 125
    Crusted cod with beans and carrots, 129
    Creamy hummus, 132
    Rich garbanzo bean spread, 133
    No-alarm Salsa, 134
    Soybean party dip, 135
    Vegetable and roquefort bean dip, 137
Beef, 57, 172
Blog, 16, 50, 187, 192

Caffeine, 28, 55–57, 65
Cancer, 12, 17, 21, 27, 33, 34, 41, 166, 167–176
Capers, 66
  recipes
    Marc's tasty tuna salad, 92
    Medley of mussels, prosciutto, and fennel on whole-wheat pasta, 114

Crusted cod with beans and carrots, 129
Carbonated beverages, 28, 37–38, 55–56
pH table, 57
Case studies, 26, 29, 35, 37, 39, 41, 47, 53, 58, 59
Celery, 46, 52
recipes
Marc's tasty tuna salad, 92
Vegetable and barley chicken soup, 101
Healthy one-pot chicken blanquette (stew), 119
Cell biology, 27, 165, 167–169
Cheese, 57, 65, 66, 67
recipes
Vegetable frittata with quinoa, 78
Quench the fire quiche with tofu and mushrooms, 82
Spinach and arugula salad with apples and pears, 89
Vegetarian sweet potato and lentil salad, 94
Prosciutto-wrapped asparagus crêpes, 96
Crisp asian chicken salad, 98
Fresh mushroom soup, 105
Scallops with penne verde, 112
Marc's kick-ass risotto with asparagus and morels, 115
Mad mushroom stew, 118
Healthy one-pot chicken blanquette (stew), 119
Vegetable and roquefort bean dip, 137
Parmesan and dill popcorn, 139
Chevalier Jackson, 161
Chicken, 26, 46, 51, 53
recipes
Crisp Asian chicken salad, 98
Vegetable and barley chicken soup, 101
Healthy one-pot chicken banquette (stew), 119
Marinated grilled chicken breast, 120
Chicken cutlet with prosciutto, 122
Chicken south-of-the-border style, 125
Chocolate, 17, 28, 55, 56, 58
Cigarettes, 28, 168
Coffee, 46, 55, 57
Conclusion, 176
Couscous, 52
recipe
Breakfast couscous with fruit and poppy seeds, 73

Dairy products, 57
butter, 55, 57
cream, 55, 57, 65
milk, 56, 62, 66
pH, 188, 189
Disclaimer, 4
Dysplasia, 41, 168

Eggs, 65, 66
Esophageal cancer, 17, 27, 37, 166, 168, 170, 176
Esophageal erosions, 13, 160
Esophagitis,13, 33, 37, 160, 164
Extraesophageal reflux disease, 13, 160

Fat content, 22, 56, 57, 65
Favorite flavorings, 65–66
Fennel, 46, 51
julienning, 114
pH, 63
recipes
Crunchy cucumber and fennel salad, 90
Medley of mussels, prosciutto, and fennel on whole-wheat pasta, 114
Food additives, 172, 173, 174–175
Food and Drug Administration (FDA), 173, 174–176
and approved practices, 173–175
Fried food, 17, 28, 35, 55, 56
Frittata, 78–79

Garlic, 59, 67
Gastric reflux, 13, 16
Gastroenterologist, 58, 159, 161, 163
Gastroenterology (GI), 26, 37, 161, 166
Gastroesophageal reflux disease (GERD), 13, 31–33, 37, 159-66
Gastro-oesophageal reflux disease (GORD) (U.K.), 13, 160
"Generally Recognized as Safe" (GRAS) standards, 174–176
Ginger, 46, 50, 67
pH, 45
recipes
Banana ginger energy smoothie, 71
Breakfast couscous with fruit and poppy seeds, 73

Crunchy cucumber and fennel salad, 90
Pearl barley and vegetable salad, 93
Asian tuna tartare, 95
Carrot and potato soup, 106
Asian pork stir-fry, 127
Spaghetti with white clam sauce, 128
No-alarm Mexican salsa, 134
Soybean party dip, 135
Pumpkin pot de crème, 143
Ginger cheesecake, 144
Ginger crêpes with bananas and cantaloupe, 149
Tropical ginger and aloe rice pudding, 150
Pear cardamom sorbet, 151
Watermelon and ginger granitè, 152
Quick banana sorbet, 153
Sweet potato and cantaloupe cake, 155
Good flavorings, 66–67
"Good Manufacturing Practices," 173–174, 176
Government Accountability Office (GAO), 174–175
Green beans, 52
pH, 64, 189
recipes
Crunchy cucumber and fennel salad, 90
Sweet potato and green bean salad, 91
Chicken cutlet with prosciutto, 122

Heartburn, 11, 13, 26, 31–33, 56, 160–161, 163–164
Hiatal hernia, 161
High-fructose corn syrup, 171–73
Hot sauce, 55, 58
pH, 64, 189
Hummus, 132

Idiosyncratic reflux foods, 51, 53, 58–59, 65
Indigestion, 7, 11, 26, 32, 175
Induction, 28
Induction diet, 45–47
Instant foods, 171–72
ISFET pH tester, 4, 16

Junk food, 171, 173

Laryngeal cancer, 27, 33, 166–169
Laryngopharyngeal reflux (LPR), 13, 26–27, 31–34, 159–170
LES "Lower Esophageal Sphincter," 28, 161, 168
Leukoplakia, 33, 168
Low-fat cooking, 65–67
Low-fat diet, 65–67
LPR, 13, 26–27, 31–34, 159–170

Melon, 45, 46, 51
pH, 63, 189
recipes
Honey, date, melon, banana, and basil crêpe, 148
Watermelon and ginger granitè, 152
Microplane, 50, 72, 73, 125, 128, 135
Mints, 35, 55, 58
Missing link, 170
Morels, 115
Mushrooms, 46, 66
pH, 63, 189
recipes
Delish mushroom omelet, 81
Quench the fire quiche with tofu and mushrooms, 82
Perfect pea soup, 104
Fresh mushroom soup, 105
Jamie's Chinese-style orzo soup, 108
Marc's kick-ass risotto with asparagus and morels, 115
Mad mushroom stew, 118
Asian pork stir-fry, 127
Soybean party dip, 135

National Soft Drink Association (NSDA), 171, 172
No-fat diet, 65
Nutrition Labeling and Information Act of 1990, 171, 173

Oatmeal, 46, 47, 50
pH, 63
recipes
OMG banana oatmeal pancakes, 74
By-the-rules oatmeal, 84
Oatmeal Marc's way, 84
Muesli-style oatmeal, 85
Crisp Asian chicken salad, 98
Oatmeal-crusted rosemary salmon, 111
Healthy one-pot chicken blanquette (stew), 119
Awesome oatmeal cookies, 141

Obesity epidemic, 22, 173
One-pot meals, 108, 116, 119
Organic foods, 53, 176
Otolaryngologist, 32, 159
Otolaryngology, 26, 161, 166

Parsley, 46, 52, 66
  pH, 63, 190
Pepper, 48, 52–53, 55
Peppers, 46, 47, 53, 55, 58, 59
  pH, 45
Pepsin, 21–25, 27, 28, 38, 40, 164, 165, 168–170, 176
  activity curve, 24
  molecule, 22
Peptic esophagitis, 13
pH monitoring, 163–164, 165, 168
pH scale, 23
  how to understand, 23
pH tables, 62–64, 188–191
Potatoes, 46
  pH, 63
  recipes
    Sweet potato and green bean salad, 91
    Vegetarian sweet potato and lentil salad, 94
    Vegetable and barley chicken soup, 101
    Carrot and potato soup, 106
    One-pot vegetable and rice tofu, 116
    Mad mushroom stew, 118
    Healthy one-pot chicken blanquette, 119
    Pork loin with fingerling potatoes and zucchini, 126
    Sweet potato bites, 136
    Sweet potato and cantaloupe cake, 155
Prosciutto
  recipes
    Prosciutto-wrapped asparagus crêpes, 96
    Perfect-pH pea soup, 102
    Medley of mussels, prosciutto, and fennel on whole-wheat pasta, 114
    Chicken cutlet with prosciutto, 122
    Rich garbanzo bean spread, 133
Proton pump inhibitors (PPI), 25, 164
  side effects, 25
Pulmonology, 166

Quinoa, 78

Reflux, 11–14
  case studies, 26, 29, 35, 37, 39, 41, 47, 53, 58, 59
  history of, 160–162
  symptoms, 32
  terms to describe, 13
Reflux diet, 27–29
Reflux laryngitis, 13, 33, 37
Reflux Symptom Index (RSI), 32
Rice, 47, 52
  recipes
    Jordan's quickie poached salmon with rosemary, 113
    Marc's kick-ass risotto with asparagus and morels, 115
    One-pot vegetable and rice tofu, 116
    Asian pork stir-fry, 127
    Asian-style shrimp with jasmine rice, 130
    Jamie's best rice with cumin and turmeric, 138
    Tropical ginger and aloe rice pudding, 150

Salsa, 134
  pH, 64, 190
Salt, 52
Seafood and fish, 52
  recipes
    Jamie's Chinese-style orzo soup, 108
    Sautéed shrimp with angel hair pasta, 110
    Oatmeal-crusted rosemary salmon, 111
    Scallops with penne verde, 112
    Jordan's quickie poached salmon with rosemary, 113
    Medley of mussels, prosciutto, and fennel on whole-wheat pasta, 114
    Crusted cod with beans and carrots, 129
    Asian-style shrimp with jasmine rice, 130
Silent reflux, see "LPR"
Sleep apnea, 33–35, 192
Sleep disorders, 34–35
Smoking, 28, 167–168
Snoring, 33–35
Soda, see "Carbonated beverages"
Soups, 100
Start-up diet, 45–47

Stomach acid, 22-23
Stricture, 33, 160
Supraesophageal reflux disease, 13, 160

Tea, 35, 38, 44, 46, 55, 57, 59, 189–190
Theobromine, 56
Three blind men, 159–61, 166
Title 21, 171, 173–174
Tobacco, 28
Tofu, 47, 53
  recipes
    Quench the fire quiche with tofu and mushrooms, 82
    One-pot vegetable and rice tofu, 116
    Soybean party dip, 135
    Ginger cheesecake, 144
    Fig and Greek yogurt on golden granola, 147
Transnasal esophagoscopy (TNE), 162, 163, 170
Tuna
  recipes
    Marc's tasty tuna salad, 92
    Asian tuna tartare, 95
Turkey, 47, 51
  recipe
    Grilled turkey breast with Japanese eggplant, 124

Vegetarian dishes
  recipes
    Banana ginger energy smoothie, 71
    Gala apple honeydew smoothie 72,
    Breakfast couscous with fruit and pine nuts, 73
    Marc's homemade 5-grain bread, 76
    By-the-rules oatmeal, 84
    Oatmeal Marc's way, 84
    Muesli-style oatmeal, 85
    Instant polenta with sesame seeds, 86
    Calm carrot salad, 88
    Spinach and arugula with apples and pears, 89
    Sweet potato and green bean salad, 91
    Pearl barley and vegetable salad (made with vegetable stock), 93
    Vegetarian sweet potato and lentil salad, 94
    Perfect-ph pea soup (made with vegetable stock), 102
    Black bean and cilantro soup, 103,
    Pea shooter with sautéed porcini (made with vegetable stock), 104
    Fresh mushroom soup (made with vegetable stock), 105,
    Carrot and potato soup (made with vegetable stock), 106
    Flavorful cantaloupe gazpacho, 107
    Jamie's Chinese-style orzo soup (made with vegetable stock), 108
    Marc's kick-ass risotto with asparagus and morels, 115
    One-pot vegetable and rice tofu, 116
    Mad mushroom stew, 118,
    Creamy hummus (made with vegetable stock), 132
Rich garbanzo bean spread, 133
No-alarm Mexican salsa, 134
Soybean party dip, 135
Sweet potato bites, 136
Vegetable and Roquefort bean dip (made with vegetable stock), 137
Jamie's best rice with cumin and turmeric, 138
Parmesan and dill popcorn, 139
Ginger cheesecake, 144
Fig and Greek yogurt on golden granola, 147
Pear cardamom sorbet, 151
Watermelon and ginger granite, 152
Quick banana sorbet, 153
Sweet potato and cantaloupe cake, 155

Water, 23, 34, 38, 44, 45, 47
Whole-grain bread, 47, 49, 50, 53

Yogurt, 66
  pH, 63, 64, 191
  recipes
    Banana ginger energy smoothie, 71
    Crunchy-wheat French toast, 75
    Healthy raisin bran muffins, 77
    Marinated grilled chicken breast, 120
    Fig and Greek yogurt on golden granola, 147